MEMORY BANK
FOR
MEDICATIONS

Second Edition

Contents

Preface

Memory Bank for Medications was written to assist nurses to increase their independent decision making regarding the dependent action of administering medications.

The idea for the book was conceived from the experience of working with students and RNs. These nurses were facing an overwhelming task—that of sorting through an immense amount of pharmaceutical data to make it into a comprehensive entity. The format of *Memory Bank for Medications* does just that; it presents the most important information on each drug and presents it in an easy-to-read way.

Memory Bank for Medications is not designed to be a prescriptive text but an informational resource. It does not include all information regarding a medication; it is intended for use as a convenient resource text. For additional information, or clarification, refer to the Physicians' Desk Reference, the manufacturer's literature, or other pharmacology texts.

The uses, doses, and other drug information presented in this publication are based on research and consultation with pharmaceutical and nursing authorities. To the best of our knowledge, this information reflects currently accepted clinical practice; nevertheless, it cannot be considered absolute. For individual application, recommendations must be considered in light of the patient's clinical condition. Before administration of new or infrequently used drugs, review of thepatient's medication profile and consultation with physician and/or the pharmacist is advised. We disclaim responsiblity for any adverse effects resulting directly or indirectly from the suggested procedures or from the reader's misunderstanding of the text.

Format Explanation

Brand Name
Selected brand names; most common one is
listed first; the others in alphabetical order.

Actions
Drug classification(s) and methods by which the
medication causes its effects; not always known.
Includes time of onset as known.

Uses
Disease processes for which the medication is
prescribed.

Contraindications
Medications, conditions, diseases with which the
medication should not be used or should be used
cautiously. When a pediatric dose is not listed,
extreme caution should be excerised if the
medication is ordered for a child.

Interactions
The most common medications that interact with
the drug.

Dose
General dosage ranges for adult and pediatric
patients; many contain recommended doses for
initial, maximum, and maintenance doses. Doses
listed are generally for the oral route; refer to
other pharmacologic resources for parental doses
not otherwise specified. Adult doses must be

individualized for older children if the medication is
not contraindicated.

Forms
Available forms of the drug.

Adverse Effects
List of common side effects that may occur.

Special Nursing Considerations and Patient Education
- General considerations for administration of the
  medication.
- What to monitor during the course of treatment
  with the medication.
- Facts relevant to patient education. Rationales
  are generally not given. Refer to other pharmacology texts for additional information.

Notice

Clinical health care is a dynamic field because of the continuous availability of new information. Eventually this new information may lead to necessary changes in treatment methodology and the use of drugs. The authors and the publisher of *Memory Bank for Medications* have carefully reviewed doses of drugs and treatment modalities for correct content and compatibility with general standards of care acceptable at the time of publication. Before administering a drug, review instructions and information on the manufacturer's package insert to verify that recommended dosage is correct and unchanged, and that no changes have occurred related to uses or contraindications of the drug. (This review is always advisable, and especially when using a new or infrequently used drug.)

Part I
Medications

Acetaminophen

Brand Name
Tylenol, Datril, Tempra

Actions
Analgesic, antipyretic; elevates pain threshold;
affects heat-regulating aspect of hypothalamus

Uses
Fever, pain

Contraindications
Anemia, glucose-6-phosphate dehydrogenase
deficiencies; cardiac or pulmonary disease

Interactions
Coumarin anticoagulants

Dose
Adult PO: 325–650 mg q4–6h to a *maximum* of 4
gm/day
Peds PO: 3–6 yr: 120 mg tid–qid
7–12 yr: 162–325 mg tid–qid

Forms
Capsules, chewable tablets, elixirs, suppositories,
tablets

Adverse Effects
Abdominal pain, nausea, vomiting; toxic doses
can cause hepatic and renal tubular necrosis

**Special Nursing Considerations
and Patient Education**
- Protect medication from direct light.
- Use as aspirin substitute to relieve pain and fever especially for patients with a viral infection.
- Be aware that
  - medication causes fewer GI adverse effects than aspirin.
  - this drug does not have anti-inflammatory effects and cannot replace aspirin in these cases.
  - it is safe at usual doses for use during lactation.

Acetazolamide

Brand Name
Diamox

Actions
Diuretic, carbonic anhydrase inhibitor (lessens
concentration of hydrogen ions in tubules). Onset
evident in 2 hours.

Uses
Chronic simple glaucoma, congestive heart
failure, convulsive disorders, edema

Contraindications
Addison's disease, chronic noncongestive angle-
closure glaucoma, hepatic disease,
hyperchloremic acidosis, low serum levels of
potassium and sodium, renal disease, supra-renal
gland disease. *Use with caution:* Past allergic
reactions to sulfa drugs, diabetes, gout, lupus
erythematosus

Interactions
Amphetamines, lithium, methenamine salts, oral
hypoglycemics, quinidine, theophylline, tricyclic
antidepressants

Dose
Adult PO: 250 mg–1 gm/day
Peds   PO: 5 mg/kg/day

Forms
Injection, sequels, tablets

Adverse Effects
Anorexia, confusion, drowsiness, hematuria, hypokalemia, paresthesia, polyuria, unusual bleeding, urticaria

Special Nursing Considerations and Patient Education
- Monitor urinary output, weight.
- Include potassium-rich foods in patient's diet (see Appendix F).
- Discontinue if electrolyte imbalance or allergic signs are evident.
- Assess edema.
- Be aware that
  - IV route is less painful than IM injection.
  - drug's effectiveness lessens after 2 days.
  - tolerance can develop.
- Teach patient
  - that medication may cause drowsiness and confusion.
  - to notify physician if tingling feeling in hands and feet, loss of appetite, fever, rash, unusual bleeding, or bruising occurs.
  - to increase fluid intake.

Acyclovir Sodium

Brand Name
Zovirax

Actions
Antiviral. Onset evident: PO unknown; IV prompt.

Uses
Genital herpes—initial treatment and management of recurrences

Contraindications
Hypersensitivity. *Use with caution:* CHF, renal disease, seizures

Interactions
Probenecid, interferon, amphoterecin, methotrexate

Dose
Adult PO: initial treatment: 200 mg q4h for a total of 5 capsules/day × 10 days; recurrences: 200 mg tid × 6 months; intermittent treatment: 200 mg q4 for a total of 5 capsules/day × 5 days; IV: 5 mg/kg q8h × 7 days; ointment: cover all lesions q3– 6 × day × 7 days

Ped IV: 250 mg/M² over 1h q8h × 7 days

Forms
Capsules, ointment, infusion

Adverse Effects
Nausea, vomiting, diarrhea, dizziness, headache,
anorexia, fatigue, edema, rash, sore throat,
medicine taste, vaginitis, moniliasis, transient
burning at application site (topical)

**Special Nursing Considerations
and Patient Education**
- Assess and monitor signs of infection.
- Administer IV: 10 ml sterile water/500 mg
  medication; use within 12 hours.
- Infuse over 1 hour.
- Initiate therapy as soon as possible after symptom
  onset.
- Provide emotional support.
- Provide educational materials.
- Teach patient to
  - contact physician if relief of symptoms and/or
    increasing recurrences occur.
  - contact physician if signs of superinfection
    occur.
  - use finger cot/gloves to apply ointment.
  - avoid contact with eyes.
  - use condoms during sexual intercourse.
  - refrain from intercourse while lesions are
    present.
  - recognize that even though symptoms are
    treated, the disease is not cured.

ALBUTEROL

Brand Name
Proventil, Ventolin

Actions
Bronchodilator, antiasthmatic. Onset evident: PO
30 minutes; inhaler 5–15 minutes.

Uses
Bronchospasm, prevention of exercise-induced
bronchospasm

Contraindications
Hypersentitivity to sympathomimetics. *Use with
caution:* Cardiac disease, hypertension,
hyperthyroidism, near-term pregnancy, diabetes

Interactions
MAO inhibitors, tricyclic antidepressants, aerosol
bronchodilators

Dose
Adult   PO: 2–3 mg tid–qid; *maxmimum dose:* 8 mg/
day; inhalation: 2 puffs q4–6h; prevention: 2
puffs prior to exercise

Forms
Tablets, aerosol, syrup

Adverse Effects
Tremors, dizziness, tachycardia, anxiety, irritation
of throat and nose, restlessness, headache,
coughing, bronchospasm, nausea, vomiting,
cardiac arrhythmias

**Special Nursing Considerations
and Patient Education**
• Monitor pulmonary function prior to administration
  and at peak of onset.
• Observe for paradoxical bronchospasm.
• Administer with meals.
• Store in light-resistant containers.
• Teach patient to
  – allow 1 minute between inhalations.
  – utilize inhaler properly.
  – not exceed prescribed dose.
  – notify physician if cardiac palpitations occur.
  – not use OTC medications.

Alcohol/Diphenhydramine HCl

Brand Name
Benylin

Actions
Antihistamine, antitussive

Uses
Cough relief

Contraindications
Meds   MAO inhibitors
Other Asthma, bladder-neck or pyloroduodenal
         obstructions, narrow-angle glaucoma,
         neonates, premature infants, prostatic
         hypertrophy, stenosing peptic ulcer. *Use with
         caution:* Asthma

Interactions
Alcohol, CNS depressants

Dose
Adult 25–50 mg tid–qid; *maximum* dose: 400 mg/
         day
Peds   5 mg/kg/day, in 4 divided doses; *maximum*
         dose: 300 mg/day

Forms
Syrup

Adverse Effects
Blurred vision, confusion, constipation, diarrhea, drowsiness, dry mouth, hypotension, nausea, nervousness, restlessness, vomiting

**Special Nursing Considerations
and Patient Education**
- Protect medication from direct light.
- Offer hard candy (regular or sugar-free) to relieve dry mouth.
- Teach patient
  - that medication may cause photosensitivity.
  - to keep syrup out of reach of children.
  - to change position slowly to decrease possibility of hypotension.
  - to be cautious when driving or involved in potentially hazardous tasks.
  - to take with meals or milk to decrease GI upset.

Allopurinol

Brand Name
Zyloprim, Lopurim

Actions
Controls hyperuricemia. Onset evident in 24–48 hours.

Uses
Gout, recurrent uric-acid stone formation, uric–acid nephropathy

Contraindications
Meds Iron preparations
Other Children (unless as an adjunct with chemotherapy), idiopathic hemochromatosis. *Use with caution:* History of hepatic or renal disease

Interactions
Anticoagulants, azathioprine, mercaptopurine, theophylline, uricosuric agents

Dose
Adult 200–600 mg/day in divided doses
Peds Under 6 yr: 50 mg tid
6-10 yr: 100 mg tid

Forms
Tablets

Adverse Effects
Alopecia, diarrhea, drowsiness, nausea, pruritus, rash, vomiting

**Special Nursing Considerations
and Patient Education**
- Give amounts of 300 mg in 1 dose.
- Reduce dose in renal failure.
- Transfer from other medications, gradually.
- Monitor blood counts, I&O, uric acid levels.
- Teach patient to
    - keep well hydrated (2,000 cc/day).
    - take each dose with full glass of water; if GI upset occurs, take with food.
    - be cautious when driving or involved in potentially hazardous tasks.
    - discontinue if rash occurs.
    - avoid large doses of Vitamin C.

Alprazolam

Brand Name
Xanax

Actions
CNS depressant. Onset evident in 1–2 hours.

Uses
Anxiety; *not* of value in treatment of psychoses

Contraindications
Meds Alcohol, hypersensitivity to benzodiazepines
Other Acute narrow-angle glaucoma, children
under 18. *Use with caution:* Hepatic or renal
impairment

Interactions
Anticonvulsants, antihistamines, barbiturates,
cimetidine, CNS depressants, hypnotics,
narcotics, oral anticoagulants, sedatives,
tranquilizers

Dose
Adult 0.25-.5 mg *tid; maximum* dose: 4 mg/day in
divide doses

Forms
Tablets

Adverse Effects
Confusion, constipation, depression, diarrhea, drowsiness, dry mouth, headache, lightheadedness, nausea, vomiting

Special Nursing Considerations and Patient Education
- Use caution when administering to patients with suicidal potential; ensure patient swallows dose.
- Monitor patient's physical and mental status periodically.
- May crush tablets.
- Provide emotional support.
- Be aware that
  - Habituation and dependence are possible; when discontinued, decrease dosage gradually.
- Teach patient
  - that effects may continue after treatment ends.
  - to be cautious when driving or involved in potentially hazardous tasks.
  - to avoid alcohol and other CNS depressants.
  - to use hard, sugar-free candy to relieve dry mouth.

Aminocaprioc Acid

Brand Name
Amicar

Actions
Fibrinolytic inhibitor, systemic hemostatic; reduces plasminogen activator substances and demonstrates antiplasmin activity

Uses
Treatment of excessive bleeding resulting from systemic hyperfibrinolysis and urinary fibrinolysis; used investigationally to prevent recurrence of subarachnoid hemorrhage

Contraindications
Active Intravascular clotting process (not used unless there is definite diagnosis of hyperfibrinolysis). *Use with caution:* Cardiac, hepatic, or renal dysfunction; uremia

Interactions
Estrogens, oral contraceptives, probenecid

Dose
Adult   PO: initial dose: 4–5 gm; then, 1–1.25 gm/hr for 8 hr or until bleeding is controlled
Peds   PO: 100 mg/kg q6h for 6 days

Forms
Injection, syrup, tablets

16

Adverse Effects

Bradycardia, dysrhythmias, hypotension (IV use); conjunctival suffusion; cramps; diarrhea; dizziness; headache; malaise; nasal stuffiness; nausea; rash; tinnitus

Special Nursing Considerations and Patient Education

- Give IV slowly, over a 30 minute period.
- Monitor Plasma levels, potassium, vital signs.
- Be aware that
  - optimal plasma level is 0.130 mg/cc.
  - medication may elevate serum potassium levels.
- Teach patient
  - to report any signs of bleeding to physician.

Aminophylline

Brand Name
Somophyllin

Actions
Bronchodilator, decongestant; inhibits phosphodiesterase which leads to increased epinephrine. Onset evident: PO 15–60 minutes; (IV) rapid.

Uses
Bronchial asthma, cardiac paroxysmal dyspnea, Cheyne-Stokes respirations, congestive heart failure, emphysema, pulmonary edema, status asthmaticus

Contraindications
Hypersensitivlty to any xanthine; rectal suppositories contraindicated in presence of irritation or Infection of rectum or lower colon. *Use with caution:* Cardiac, hepatic, or renal dysfunction; coronary artery disease; hypertension; hyperthyroid; MI; peptic ulcer; porphyria; prostatic hypertrophy

Interactions
Beta-blocking agents, tetracycline, reserpine, chlordiazepoxide; *effects decreased* by cigarette smoke, phenobarbital; *effects increased by* allopurinol cimetidine, clindamycin, influenza

18

vaccine, lincomycin, thiabendazole; *increases* effects of adrenergics, digitalis, furosemide, oral anticoagulants; *decreases* effects of lithium, phenytoin. Medication is incompatible with many IV drugs.

Dose
Adult   PO: 100–315 mg q6–8h
Peds   PO: 3.5–5 mg/kg q6–8h

Forms
Elixir, extended-action tablets, injection, oral liquid, rectal solution, suppository, tablets

Adverse Effects
Diarrhea, dizziness, extrasystoles, flushing, generalized convulsions, headache, hypotension, irritability, nausea, palpitations, restlessness, tachypnea, vomiting

Special Nursing Considerations and Patient Education
• Warm IV solutions to body temperature, dilute, give slowly.
• Give oral forms with glass of water on an empty stomach 1 hour before or 2 hours after meals.
• Do not administer with food.
• Administer on a regular basis over 24 hours.
• Monitor vital signs.
• Maintain plasma levels at 10–20 μg/cc.
• Be aware that
  – IM injection is very painful.

- Teach patient
  - to be cautious when driving or involved in potentially hazardous tasks.
  - to notify physician of cramps, dizziness, headache, insomnia, palpitations, stomach upset.
  - that smoking may decrease effectiveness of medication.
  - to retain rectal dose for 20–30 minutes.

Notes

_____

_____

_____

_____

_____

_____

_____

_____

_____

_____

_____

_____

_____

_____

_____

_____

Aminosalicylic Acid
(Para-Aminosalicylic Acid)

Brand Name
PAS

Actions
Antitubercular, bacteriostatic; delays tubercle resistance to isoniazid and streptomycin

Uses
Adjunct in treatment of extrapulmonary and pulmonary tuberculosis

Contraindications
Med   Salicylates
Other   Renal dysfunction. *Use with caution:* Peptic ulcer

Interactions
Ammonium chloride, digitalis, isoniazid, oral anticoagulants, phenytoin, probenecid, pyrazinamide, rifampin

Dose
Adult   8–15 gm/day in 2–4 equal doses
Peds   200–300 mg/kg/day in equal doses

Forms

Buffered tablets, enteric-coated tablets, resins,
tablets, solutions

Adverse Effects
Abdominal pain, acidosis, agranulocytosis,
anorexia, diarrhea, eosinophilia, hypokalemia,
leukopenia, nausea, rash, vomiting

**Special Nursing Considerations
and Patient Education**
• Teach patient
  – to store medication away from moisture.
  – to use oral solutions within 24 hours.
  – to discard medication if it has brown or purple
    coloring.
  – to use Tes-Tape to test urine of diabetic patient.
  – that medication may cause a peculiar taste in
    mouth.
  – to keep well hydrated.
  – to avoid medications or foods that acidify urine
    (e.g., cranberry juice).
  – to take oral forms after meals to help decrease
    GI distress.
  – that medication may cause abnormal
    discoloration of urine.
  – to discontinue medication for unusual bleeding,
    fever, rash, sore throat, peculiar taste in mouth.

Amitriptyline HCl

Brand Name
Elavil, Endep, Etrafon

Actions
Tricyclic antidepressant; affects central nervous system. Onset evident in 1–2 weeks.

Uses
Depression, enuresis (children)

Contraindications
Meds   Alcohol, ethchlorvynol, MAO inhibitors, procainamide, quinidine, reserpine, thyroid preparations
Other   Closed-angle glaucoma, MI, prostatic hypertrophy, pyloric stenosis, renal dysfunction, urinary retention. *Use with caution:* Asthma, diabetes, epilepsy, GI and hepatic disorders

Interactions
Adrenergics, amphetamines, anticholinergics, anticonvulsants, antihistamines, beta-blockers, clonidine, CNS depressants, guanethidine, levodopa, narcotics, oral coumarins, sedatives, tranquilizers dysfunction, hyperthyroidism

Dose

Adult   PO: 10–25 mg bid–qid (hospitalized patients
        may need as much as 300 mg/day)
Peds   PO: Adolescent: 10 mg tid with 20 mg at hs

Forms
  Injection, tablets

Adverse Effects
Anorexia, blurred vision, dizziness, drowsiness, dry
        mouth, headache, nausea, peculiar taste,
        orthostatic hypotension, vomiting

**Special Nursing Considerations
and Patient Education**
• Administer with meals.
• Offer hard, sugar-free candy to relieve dry mouth.
• Provide emotional support.
• Decrease dosage slowly.
• Teach patient
    – that medicine may cause urine to be colored
      blue-green, and may cause photosensitivity.
    – to be cautious when driving or involved in
      potentially hazardous tasks.
    – not to take other medications without consulting
      with physician.
    – to avoid alcohol.
    – to change positions slowly.
    – that therapeutic effects may take 1–2 weeks.

Amobarbital, Amobarbital Sodium

Brand Name
   Amytal, Tuinal

Actions
   Hypnotic, sedative, barbiturate. Onset evident in
   30–60 minutes.

Uses
   Acute convulsive disorders, insomnia

Contraindications
Meds Alcohol, CNS depressants
Other History of porphyria; renal dysfunction;
          uncontrolled pain. *Use with caution:* Asthma,
          borderline hypoadrenalism, cardiac
          dysfunction, hepatic or pulmonary
          dysfuntion, hypertension (IM/IV use),
          hypotension, hypothyroidism, respiratory
          distress

Interactions
   Antidepressants, beta-blockers, cortisone,
   digitalis, griseofulvin, MAO inhibitors, narcotics,
   oral anticoagulants, oral contraceptives,
   phenylbutazone, phenytoin, quinidine,
   tetracycline, valproic acid

Dose

Adult PO: Hypnotic: 100–200 mg; sedative: 30–50
mg bid–tid
Peds PO: 3–6 mg/kg/day in 3 equal doses

Forms
Capsules, elixir, sodium salt injection, tablets

Adverse Effects
Ataxia, dizziness, emotional disturbances,
excitement, lethargy, nausea, pruritus,
restlessness

**Special Nursing Considerations
and Patient Education**
- Medication is addictive; when discontinued,
  decrease dosage gradually.
- Inject IM doses into deep muscle; give no more
  than 5 cc at one site.
- Monitor vital signs closely when giving IV;
  maximum IV rate is 1 cc/minute.
- When used as a hypnotic, administer 30–60
  minutes before hs.
- Provide safety measures.
- Teach patient
  - that medication can lower body temperature; if
    elderly, to be cautious during cold weather.
  - that medication may cause photosensitivity.
  - to be cautious when driving or involved in
    potentially hazardous tasks.
  - to avoid alcohol or CNS depressants.
  - that medication is for short-term use only.
  - to use alternate methods of relaxation.

AMOXICILLIN

Brand Name
Amoxil, Trimox, Larotid, Polymox, Sumox,
Ultimox, Wymox

Actions
Antibiotic; bactericidal; inhibits synthesis of cell
wall of sensitive organisms

Uses
Infections—hemophilus, H. influenzae, E. coli, P.
mirabilis, N. gonorrhoeae, streptococci

Contraindications
Use with caution: hypersensitivity to penicillins.

Interactions
Probenecid, aspirin, tetracycline, erythromycin

Dose
Adult   PO: 250 mg–500 mg q8h
Peds   PO: 20–40 mg/kg/day in divided doses q8h

Forms
Capsules, chewable tablets, powder for oral
suspension, pediatric drops

Adverse Effects

Anemia, diarrhea, furry tongue, nausea, rashes, sore mouth, vomiting

Special Nursing Considerations and Patient Education

- Administer oral form around the clock (absorption not significantly affected by food presence).
- Teach patient to
  - complete full course of therapy.
  - to report signs of superinfection (e.g., furry tongue, diarrhea, or rash).
  - carry Medic Alert card or bracelet if allergic to penicillin.

Amoxicillin/Clavulanate Potassium

Brand Name
Augmentin

Actions
Broad spectrum antibiotic. Rapid onset.

Uses
Sinus infection, lower respiratory infection, otitus media, skin and skin structure infection, genitourinary tract infection, meningitis, septicemia. Effective against: E. coli, H. influenzae, P. mirabilis, salmonella

Contraindications
Hypersensitivity to penicillin.

Interactions
Aspirin, probenecid, tetracyclines, erythromycins

Dose
Adult: PO: 250–500 mg q8h
Peds: PO: 20–40 mg/kg/day in divided doses

Forms
Tablets, chewable, powder for oral suspension

Adverse Effects
Nausea and vomiting, vaginitis,moniliasis, diarrhea, rashes, superinfections, urticaria

Special Nursing Considerations and Patient Education
- Provide adequate fluid intake.
- Administer in equal doses around the clock.
- Observe for signs and symptoms of anaphylaxis.
- Teach patient to
  - complete full course of treatment.
  - notify physician if diarrhea or sore throat occur.
  - take around the clock.

Ampicillin, Ampicillin Sodium

Brand Name
Polycillin, Amcill, Omnipen, SK-Ampicillin

Actions
Interferes with ability of susceptible bacteria to create cell walls as they multiply and grow

Uses
Endocarditis; meningitis; respiratory tract, skin, soft tissue, and urinary tract infections

Contraindications
Meds Hypersensitivity to penicillins or cephalosporins
Other Infectious mononucleosis. *Use with caution:* Renal failure

Interactions
Bacteriostatic antibiotics (erythromycin, tetracycline), oral contraceptives, probenecid

Dose
Adult PO: 250–500 mg q6h
Peds PO: 25–50 mg/kg/day in divided doses q6–8h

Forms
Chewable tablets, pediatric drops, sodium salt injection, trihydrate capsules or suspension

Adverse Effects
Dark discoloration of tongue, diarrhea, glossitis,
nausea, nephritis, stomatitis, superinfections,
urticaria

**Special Nursing Considerations
and Patient Education**
- Refrigerate liquid forms.
- Inject IV form slowly (2 cc /3–5 minutes).
- Monitor urinary output.
- Administer oral forms 1 hour before or 2 hours
  after meals.
- If an outpatient, have patient remain in office for
  30 minutes after receiving medication for first
  time.
- Inspect skin frequently tor signs of rash.
- Be aware that
  - a cross reaction is possible it patient is
    hypersensitive to cephalosporins.
- Teach patient to
  - take entire prescription.
  - notify physician if signs of superinfection occur
    (e.g., tarry stools, black tongue).

Amyl Nitrite

Actions
Antianginal, coronary vasodilator. Onset evident in 30 seconds.

Uses
Angina pectoris, antidote for cyanide poisoning

Contraindications
Cerebral hemorrhage, head trauma

Interactions
Alcohol, antihypertensive narcotics, tricyclics

Dose
Adult   0.18–0.3 cc prn

Forms
Inhaler

Adverse Effects

Flushing, headache, hypotension, nausea, reflex
tachycardia, syncope, vomiting

**Special Nursing Considerations
and Patient Education**
- Be aware that
  - medication has strong, unpleasant odor.
- Teach patient
  - that medication is flammable.
  - correct usage of inhaler: sit down and take deep
    breaths.
  - to monitor angina attacks; keep journal.
  - to change position slowly.

Aspirin

Brand Name
ASA, Ecotrin, Empirin

Actions
Analgesic (raises pain threshold), anti-inflammatory, antipyretic (affects heat-regulatory center of hypothalamus). Onset evident in 15–20 minutes.

Uses
Fever, relief of mild to moderate pain, rheumatic fever, rheumatoid arthritis

Contraindications
Meds   Anticoagulants, ulcerogenics
Other   Active ulcers, tendency to hemorrhage. *Use with caution:* Anemia, asthma, diabetes, hepatic or renal dysfunction, history of ulcers or gout, Hodgkin's disease, hypoprothrombinemia, viral infection

Interactions
Alcohol, antacids, furosemide, methotrexate, oral anticoagulants, phenylbutazone, probenecid, spironolactone, steroids, sulfinpyrazone, urinary acidifiers

Dose

Adult PO: 325–650 mg q3–4h
Peds PO: 65 mg/kg/day in divided doses q6h

Forms
Capsules, children's tablets, enteric-coated
tablets, suppository tablets

Adverse Effects
Asthma, GI bleeding, indigestion, nausea, tarry
stools, vomiting

**Special Nursing Considerations
and Patient Education**
- Do not administer if it has a vinegar odor.
- If stomach upset occurs, try a different brand.
- Be aware that
  - medication may cause false positive
    urineglucose tests.
  - aspirin should not be given to patients with a
    viral infection (may lead to Reye's syndrome).
- Teach patient to
  - assess aspirin content of other current
    medications.
  - notify physician of ringing in ears or persistent
    GI pain.
  - keep out of reach of children.
  - take with full glass of water or milk.

Aspirin/Butalbital/Caffeine

Brand Name
Fiorinal

Actions
Analgesic, antipyretic

Uses
Tension headache

Contraindications
Children under 12, porphyria. *Use with caution:*
Coagulation disorders, peptic ulcer, viral
infections.

Interactions
Alcohol, hypnotics, sedatives

Dose
Adult 1–2 tablets q4h; *maximum* dose: 6 tablets/
day

Forms
Tablets

Adverse Effects
Dizziness, drowsiness, GI distress, lightheadedness

**Special Nursing Considerations
and Patient Education**
- Administer with meals to decrease irritation.
- When discontinued, decrease dosage gradually.
- Be aware that
- dependence is possible.
- Teach patient
  - to be cautious when driving or involved in
    potentially hazardous tasks.

Aspirin/Caffeine/
Orphenadrine Citrate

Brand Name
Norgesic, Norgestic Forte

Actions
Skeletal muscle relaxant

Uses
Acute painful musculoskeletal conditions,
parkinsonism

Contraindications
Achalasia, cardiospasm, glaucoma, intestinal
obstruction, myasthenia gravis, urinary retention;
children under 12. *Use with caution:* Renal
disorders, tachycardia, viral infections

Interactions
Alcohol, CNS depressants

Dose
Adult   ½–2 tablets tid–qid

Forms
Tablets

Adverse Effects

Blurred vision, constipation, dizziness, drowsiness, dry mouth, headache, increased ocular tension, nausea, nephrotoxicity, palpitation, pruritus, pupil dilation, tachycardia, vomiting

Special Nursing Considerations and Patient Education

- Offer hard candy (regular or sugar-free) to relieve dry mouth.
- Increase fluid and bulk intake to help relieve constipation.
- Teach Patient
  - to be cautious when driving or involved in potentially hazardous task.

Atenolol

Brand Name
Tenormin

Actions
Antihypertensive; beta-adrenergic blocking agent.
Onset evident in 60 minutes.

Uses
Mild-moderate hypertension, migraines, angina
pectoris

Contraindications
Sinus bradycardial, cardiogenic shock, overt
cardiac failure, heart block greater than first
degree, pulmonary edema. *Use with caution:*
asthma, emphysema, nursing mothers, pregnancy

Interactions
IV phenytoin, verapamil, general anesthesia,
digitalis, insulin, theophyllines, antocholinergics,
sympathicomimetics

Dose
Adult PO: 50 mg qd; may increase to 100 mg
after 1–2 weeks

Forms
Tablets

Adverse Effects
Bradycardia, bronchospasm, hypotension, fatigue, mental changes, dizziness, hyper- or hypoglycemia, GI difficulties, rash, impotence

Special Nursing Considerations and Patient Education
- Administer before meals and hs.
- Monitor vital signs every 4 hours; hold if pulse is less than 50.
- Provide safety measures as indicated.
- Provide small frequent meals.
- Evaluate edema.
- Store in light-resistant containers.
- Monitor I&O, weight (signs and symptoms of congestive heart failure).
- Teach the patient to
  - not discontinue medication abruptly.
  - not use OTC medications.
  - monitor pulse.
  - avoid alcohol.
  - report any central nervous system effects.
  - avoid driving.
  - monitor serum glucose (if diabetic).

Atropine Sulfate

Actions
Anticholinergic, antispasmodic, mydriatic. Onset evident in 1–2 hours.

Uses
Bradycardia, bronchial asthma, cardiospasm, colitis, dysmenorrhea, enuresis, GI spasm, paralysis agitans, parkinsonism, pylorospasm, rigid/spastic conditions caused by CNS injury, ureteral colic, urinary frequency

Contraindications
Adhesions between iris and lens, hepatic or renal dysfunction, intestinal atony, myasthenia gravis, narrow-angle glaucoma, obstructive conditions of GI and urinary tract, reflex esophagitis, ulcerative colitis. *Use with caution:* Angina, chronic bronchitis, debilitated patients with chronic lung disease, hiatal hernia, prostatic hypertrophy, tachycardia

Interactions
Antacids, anticholinergics, antihistamines, guanethidine, haloperidol, MAO inhibitors, methylphenidate, nitrates, primidone, procainamide, quinidine, reserpine

Dose
Adult PO: 0.4–0.6 mg q4–6h
Peds   PO: 0.01 mg/kg q4–6h

Forms
Injection, ophthalmic ointment or solution, tablets

Adverse Effects
Blurred vision, constipation, cycloplegia, dry
mouth, flushing, increased intraocular pressure,
mydriasis, nausea, suppression of body
secretions, vomiting

**Special Nursing Considerations
and Patient Education**
- Store in light-resistant containers.
- Monitor vital signs.
- Offer hard candy (regular or sugar-free) to relieve
  dry mouth.
- Provide increased fluids and bulk in diet to ease
  constipation.
- Administer tablets 30 minutes before meals.
- Discontinue for eye pain, flushing, rash.
- Teach patient
  - to avoid strenuous work in hot weather to
    prevent heat stroke.
  - to be cautious when driving or involved in
    potentially hazardous tasks.
  - to report changes in vision.
  - proper instillation technique.

Benztropine Mesylate

Brand Name
Cogentin

Actions
Anticholinergic; hinders synaptic transmissions in cholinergic neurons In CNS. Onset evident in 2–3 days.

Uses
Adjunct therapy of all forms of parkinsonism; used in control of extrapyramidal disorders (except tardive dyskinesia) resulting from neuroleptic drugs (e.g., phenothiazines)

Contraindications
Meds Alcohol, nonprescription cough/hay fever preparations
Other Children under 3, closed-angle glaucoma. *Use with caution:* Atropine sensitivity, cardiovascular disease, children over 3, glaucoma, hepatic or renal dysfunction, hypertension, hyperthyroid, intestinal atony or obstruction, myasthenia gravis, prostatic hypertrophy, respiratory problems, tachycardia, ulcerative colitis, urinary retention

Interactions
Mantadine, antidiarrheals, antihistamines, antimuscarinics, CNS depressants, cortisone, haloperidol, levodopa, meperidine, methyl-phenidate, orphenadrine, phenothiazines, primidone, procainamide, quinidine, tranquilizers, tricyclic antidepressants

Dose
Adult 0.5–6 mg/day; therapy should be initiated
with a low dose and increased gradually at 5
or 6 day intervals
Peds Lower dose than adult; individualized

Forms
Injection, tablets

Adverse Effects
Blurred vision, constipation, difficult urination,
dizziness, dry mouth, mydriasis, sedation, toxic
psychosis, vomiting, weakness

**Special Nursing Considerations
and Patient Education**
- Store in light-resistant container.
- Monitor for fine vermicular tongue movements
(may indicate early tardive dyskinesia).
- Administer after meal to aid in reduction of
stomach upset.
- When discontinued, decrease dose gradually.
- Offer hard candy (regular or sugar-free) to relieve
dry mouth.
- Monitor I&O.
- Be aware that
  – IM, IV, and oral doses are the same.
  – medication is cumulative; has abuse potential.
- Teach patient to
  – avoid alcohol and other CNS depressants.
  – be cautious when driving or involved in
potentially hazardous tasks.
  – avoid strenuous activity in hot weather to
prevent heat stroke.
  – notify physician if having eye pain, taking
antipsychotics, experiencing GI complications.   4

Betaxolo Hydrochloride

Brand Name
Betoptic

Actions
Antiglaucoma; beta-adrenergic blocking agent

Uses
Chronic open-angle glaucoma, ocular
hypertension

Contraindications
Sinus bradycardia, greater than first degree AV
block, cardiagenic shock, overt cardiac failure.
Use with caution: diabetes, reactive airway
disease

Interactions
Epinephrine, reserpine, adrenergic psychotropics

Doses
Adult   One drop in affected eye bid

Forms
Sterile opthalmic solution

Adverse Effects
Tearing, brief ocular discomfort, corneal
sensitivity, itching sensation, keratitis, photophobia

**Special Nursing Considerations
and Patient Education**
- Teach patient to
  - properly instill drops.
  - wear sunglasses as needed.

Bumetanide

Brand Name
Bumex

Actions
Diuretic, antihypertensive. Onset evident: PO 30–60 minutes; IM 40 minutes; IV rapid.

Uses
Edema associated with CHF, renal and hepatic disease, pulmonary edema, nephrotic syndrome, hypertension

Contraindications
Anuria, hypovalemia, hepatic coma. *Use with caution:* diabetes, electrolyte depletion, severe liver disease

Interactions
Lithium, probenecid, indomethacin, antihypertensives, aminoglycosides

Doses
Adult   PO: 0.5–2.0 mg as single dose, may give 2nd or 3rd dose q4–5h; *maximum* dose: 10 mg/day; may give on alternate days. IM/IV: 0.5–1 mg q2–3h; *maximum* dose: 10 mg/day

Forms
Injection, tablets

Adverse Effects
Muscle cramps, dizziness, hypotension,
headache, nausea, impaired hearing, pruritis,
rash, hyperglycemia, metabolic alkalosis,
dehydration, hyperuricemia, hypochloremia,
hypokalemia, azotemia, hyponatremia.

**Special Nursing Considerations
and Patient Education**
* Monitor electrolytes prior to and during therapy.
* Monitor blood pressure and apical pulse prior to
  and during administration.
* Monitor weight, I and O.
* Assess for hearing loss.
* Administer with food to decrease GI discomfort.
* Administer IV over 1–2 minutes.
* Administer in early AM.
* Use reconstituted solution within 24 hours.
* Reconstitute with 5% dextrose/water, 0.9% NaCl
  or Lactated Ringers.
* Assess edema—abdominal girth, urinary output.
* Teach patient to
  – change position slowly.
  – follow high-potassium diet.

Buspirone Hydrochloride

Brand Name
Buspar

Actions
Antianxiety

Uses
Management of anxiety disorders, short-term
relief of anxiety symptoms

Contraindications
Hypersensitivity children, severe renal or hepatic
impairment

Interactions
MAO inhibitors, psychotrapic medications,
alcohol, trazodone, digoxin

Doses
Adult: PO: 5 mg tid; may increase 5 mg/day every
2–3 days; *maximum* dose: 60 mg/day

Forms
Tablets

Adverse Effects
Dizziness, drowsinessg nervousness, insomnia,
lightheadedness, nausea, dry mouth, numbness,
headache, fatigue, weakness, nonspecific chest
pain, sore throat, nasal congestions cardiac
disturbances

**Special Nursing Considerations
and Patient Education**
- Monitor blood pressure.
- Offer sugar-free, hard candy to relieve dry mouth.
- Assess mental status.
- Administer with food to decrease GI discomfort.
- Provide safety measures.
- Provide supportive care regarding anxiety.
- Teach patient to
    - notify physician if preganancy is suspected
    - avoid alcohol, OTC medications.
    - not take for longer than four months unless ordered by physician.
    - be aware that therapeutic effects may take 1–2 weeks.
    - not discontinue medication abruptly.

Butabarbital Sodium

Brand Name
Butisol

Actions
Depresses sensory cortex; decreases motor activity; alters cerebellar function; produces drowsiness, sedation, and hypnosis. Onset evident in 5–30 minutes.

Uses
Hypnotic, sedative, barbiturate

Contraindications
Meds Alcohol, CNS depressants
Other Hepatic dysfunction, porphyria. *Use with caution:* Acute or chronic pain; cardio-vascular, hepatic or renal dysfunction; hypertension; hypoadrenalism; hypotension; narrow-angle glaucoma; respiratory distress

Interactions
Analgesics; anticonvulsants; antidepressants; antihistamines; barbiturates; corticosterolds; digitalis; digitoxin; doxycycline; griseofulvin; hypnotics; isoniazid; MAO inhibitors; narcotics; oral anticoagulants, antidiabetics, or contraceptives; phenylbutazone; sedatives; tranquilizers

54

Dose

Adult Hypnotic: 50–100 mg hs PO; sedative: 15–
30 mg tid–qid PO

Peds 6 mg/kg/day in 3 divided doses

Forms

Capsules, elixir, extended-action tablets, tablets

Adverse Effects

Bradycardia, diarrhea, dizziness, drowsiness,
emotional problems, excitement, hypotension,
nausea, respiratory depression, vomiting

**Special Nursing Considerations
and Patient Education**

- Protect elixir from light.
- Reduce dosage for elderly or debilitated patients
  because of possibility of increased sensitivity.
- When discontinued, decrease dosage gradually.
- Administer 30–60 minutes before hs.
- Monitor respiratory status.
- Be aware that
  - medication induces hepatic microsomal
    enzymes, resulting in increased metabolism of
    many drugs.
  - medication is addictive.
- Teach patient to
  - be cautious when driving or involved in
    potentially hazardous tasks.
  - be cautious during cold weather (medication
    may substantially decrease body temperature).
  - avoid alcohol and other CNS depressants.

Captopril

Brand Name
Capoten

Actions
Antihypertensive; angiotensin-converting enzyme inhibitor. Rapid onset.

Uses
Hypertension, congestive heart failure

Contraindications
Hypersensitivity. *Use with cautions:* dialysis patients, renal diseases, patients an diuretics, diabetes mellitus, lupus erythematosis, scleroderma, COPD, asthma, aortic stenosis, cardiac insufficiency

Interactions
Diuretics, antihypertensives, vasodilators, potassium-sparing diuretics, prozosin, adrenergic blockers

Dose

Adult   PO: hypertension: initial dose: 25 mg bid–tid then 50 mg bid–tid; average dose: 25–150 mg bid–tid; *maximum* dose: 450 mg/day; congestive heart failure: 6.25–25 mg tid; *maximum* dose: 450 mg/day

Forms
Tablets

Adverse Effects
Rash, taste impairment, hypotension, tachycardia, dizziness, proteinuria, urinary frequency, photosensitivity, anorexia, GI irritation, Raynaud's Syndrome, mouth sores

**Special Nursing Considerations
and Patient Education**
- Monitor blood pressure during initial administration.
- Weigh every day if on diuretics concurrently.
- Assess urine protein.
- Administer 1 hour before or 2 hours after meals.
- Inform the patient that taste impairment is reversible (8–12 weeks).
- Teach the patient to
  - avoid sudden changes in position.
  - not discontinue the medication abruptly.
  - use sunscreen.
  - notify physician if edema or chest pain occur.
  - utilize good oral hygiene.
  - avoid OTC medications.

Carbamazepine

Brand Name
  Tegretol

Actions
  Analgesic, anticonvulsant. Onset evident in 2–4
  days.

Uses
  Glossopharyngeal or trigeminal neuraglia; grand
  mal, mixed, or partial seizures

Contraindications
Meds   MAO inhibitors
Other   Bone-marrow depression, hypersensitivity
           to tricyclic antidepressants. *Use with caution:*
           Cardiovascular, hepatic, or renal
           dysfunction; increased intraocular pressure

Interactions
  Doxycycline, oral anticoagulants or
  contraceptives, troleandomycin

Dose
Adult   Initial Dose: 200 mg/day; increase by 200
           mg/day until best response is obtained;
           maximum recommended dose: 1,200 mg/
           day (up to 1,600 mg/day has been used in
           rare instances)
Peds   10–20 mg/kg/day

Forms
  Tablets

Adverse Effects
  Blood dyscraslas, confusion, congestive heart
  failure, dizziness, drowsiness, headache, leg
  cramps, nausea, unsteadiness, urinary retention,
  vomiting

**Special Nursing Considerations
and Patient Education**
• Monitor blood results (for dyscraslas), I&O, vital
  signs.
• When discontinued, decrease dosage gradually.
• If patient has tic douloureux, help identify
  behaviors that seem to provoke attacks.
• Administer with food to avoid GI upset.
• Teach patient to
  – be cautious when driving or involved in
    potentially hazardous tasks.
  – notify physician if fever, purpuric hemorrhage,
    sore throat, or oral ulcers occur.
  – Use alternative form of contraceptive.

Cefaclor

Brand Name
Ceclor

Actions
Antibiotic. Onset rapid.

Uses
Upper and lower respiratory tract infection, otitis media urinary tract infection, dermatological infection

Contraindications
Hypersensitivity to cephalosporins or penicillin; infants under 1 month

Interactions
Tetracyclines, erythromycins, probenecid, aminoglycosides, alcohol

Dose
Adult PO: 250–500 mg q8h
Peds PO: 20–40 mg/kg/day in divided doses q8h; *maximum* dose: 1 g/day

Forms
Capsules, oral suspensions

Adverse Effects
   Abdominal pain, anorexia, diarrhea, dizziness,
   headache, nausea, rashes, superinfections (e.g.,
   black tongue, vaginal irritations)

**Special Nursing Considerations
and Patient Education**
- Administer with food to decrease GI problems.
- Check alcohol content of other medications
  patient is also taking (may cause desulfiran-type
  reaction).
- Suspension must be refrigerated.
- Monitor bowel pattern.
- Discard suspension after 14 days.
- Teach the patient to
   - take all medications as ordered.
   - inform physician if signs of superinfection occur.
   - take yogurt or buttermilk to ease diarrhea.

Cefuroxime Axetil

Brand Name
Ceftin

Actions
Broad spectrum antibiotic

Uses
Treatment of pharyngitis and tonsilitis caused by Spyogenes, otitis media caused by Spneumoniae, H. influenzae, B. catarrhalis, S. pyogenes; lower respiratory tract infections caused by S. pneumoniae, H. influenzae; urinary tract infections caused by E. coli, K. pneumonae and skin and skin structure infections caused by S. aureus, S. pyogenes

Contraindications
Hypersensitivity to cephalosporins. *Use with caution:* allergy to penicillin

Interactions
Tetracyclines, erythromycin, furosemide, probenecid.

Dose
Adult   Over 12 yr: PO: 250 mg bid; may increase to 500 mg bid; UTI: 125 mg bid; may increase to 250 mg bid
PEDS   125 mg bid

Forms
Tablets

Adverse Effects
Nausea, vomiting, diarrhea, vaginitis, rash,
pruritis, urticaria, headache

**Special Nursing Considerations
and Patient Education**
- Administer tablet whole; have patient swallow
  whole (bitter taste).
- Administer with food to decrease GI discomfort.
- Monitor urine for C & S prn.
- Observe for signs and symptoms of allergic
  reaction— rash, chills, fever, joint pain, pruritis.
- Teach patient to
  - swallow tablet whole.
  - take all the prescribed medication.
  - eat yogurt to maintain intestinal flora.

Cephalexin

Brand Name
Keflex

Actions
Antibiotic (cephalosporin); impedes synthesis of mucopeptide cell walls. Rapid onset.

Uses
Infections of respiratory tract, skin and soft tissue, urinary tract

Contraindications
Hypersensitivity to cephalosporin anibiotics. *Use with caution:* allergy to penicillin, renal dysfunction

Interactions
Concomitant use with nephrotoxic agent (aminoglycosides) increases probability of nephrotoxicity; probenecid

Dose
Adult   250–500 mg q6h
Peds   Over 1 month of age: 25–50 mg/kg/day in 4 divided dose

Forms
Capsule, pediatric drops, suspension, tablets

Adverse Effects
Blood dyscrasias, diarrhea, dizziness, drowsiness, dyspepsia, headache, nausea, pseudomembranous colitis, rash, urticaria, vomiting

Special Nursing Considerations and Patient Education
- Refrigerate solutions and discard unused portion after 2 weeks.
- Monitor for nonsusceptible microbe overgrowth.
- Use Clintest or Tes-Tape to test urine for sugar.
- Discontinue if diarrhea or rash occurs.
- Monitor for signs of anaphylaxis.
- Monitor I&O.
- May administer with food to decrease GI irritation.
- Monitor IV for phlebitis.
- Be aware that
  - sensitivity to penicillin may occur.
  - medication may cause false-positive Coombs' test and glycosuria.
- Teach patient to
  - complete full course of therapy.
  - report signs of superinfection (e.g., black tongue, itching).

Chloral Hydrate

Brand Name
Noctec

Actions
Hypnotic, sedative. Onset evident in 30–60 minutes.

Uses
Delirium tremens, hypnotic, sedative, withdrawal from barbiturates or narcotics

Contraindications
Meds   Alcohol, CNS depressants
Other   Cardiac, hepatic, or renal dysfunction; gastric ulcer; gastritis. *Use with caution:* Colitis, depression, drug abusers, proctitis

Interactions
Antihistamines, barbiturates, furosemide, hypnotics, MAO inhibitors, narcotics, oral anticoagulants, phenothiazines, sedatives, tranquilizers, tricyclic antidepressants

Dose
Adult   PO: Hypnotic: 0.5–1 gm; sedative: 250 mg tid
Peds   PO: Hypnotic: 50 mg/kg; *maximum* dose: 1 gm; sedative: 25 mg/kg/day In 3–4 divided doses

Forms
Capsules, elixir, suppository, syrup

Adverse Effects
Confusion, dizziness, drowsiness, gastritis, hallucinations, headache, nausea, paradoxical behavior, peculiar taste, vomiting

Special Nursing Considerations and Patient Education
- Refrigerate suppositories.
- Use caution when administering to patients with suicidal potential; ensure patient swallows dose.
- Mix liquid forms in a glass of fruit juice, ginger ale, or water.
- When used as a hypnotic, administer 15–30 minutes prior to hs.
- When discontinued, decrease dosage gradually.
- Administer on empty stomach if possible.
- Do not crush or chew.
- Be aware that
  – tolerance or addiction can develop.
- Teach patients to
  – be cautious when driving or involved in potentially hazardous tasks.
  – avoid alcohol and other CNS depressants.
  – use alternate methods of relaxation.

Chlordiazepoxide HCl

Brand Name
Librium, A-poxide, Libritabs

Actions
Depression of limbic system of CNS and reticular
formation of brainstem. Onset evident: PO: 30–60
minutes; IM 15–30 minutes; IV 3–30 minutes.

Uses
Alcohol withdrawal, anticonvulsant, muscle
relaxant, tranquilizer

Contraindications
Meds Alcohol, hypersensitivity to benzodiazepines
Other Acute intermittent porphyria, acute narrow-
angle glaucoma, children under 12,
myasthenia gravis. *Use with caution:*
Emphysema; hepatic, pulmonary, or renal
dysfunction

Interactions
Anticonvulsants, antihistamines, barbiturates,
cimetidine, CNS depressants, hypnotics,
narcotics, oral contraceptives, oral anticoagulants,
sedatives, tranquilizers

Dose
Adult PO: 5–25 mg bid–qid
Peds PO: Over 6 yr: 5 mg bid–qid

Forms
Capsules, injection, tablets

Adverse Effects
Ataxia, confusion, constipation, depression, dizziness, drowsiness, extrapyramidal symptons, headache, lethargy, orthostatic hypotension

Special Nursing Considerations and Patient Education
- Store medication in light-resistant containers.
- When discontinued, decrease dose gradually.
- When administering IM/IV, follow dispensing directions carefully. Use only diluent provided in package.
- Give IV dose slowly over at least 1 minute.
- Monitor I&O until drug dosage is stable.
- Monitor blood counts and liver function if therapy is continued over extended period of time.
- May crush tablets.
- Do not take for longer than 4 months without physician's order.
- Be aware that
  - medication can be addictive and cumulative.
  - IM absorption is poor.
- Teach patient
  - to avoid prolonged exposure to sunlight since photosensitivity may occur.
  - that smoking may decrease effectiveness of medication.
  - to be cautious when driving or involved in potentially hazardous tasks.
  - to decrease caffeine intake because of its stimulant effects.
  - to notify physician for unusual bleeding, fever, sore throat.
  - to avoid alcohol and other CNS depressants.
  - to avoid OTC medications.
  - to change position slowly.

Chlorothiazide

Brand Name
Diuril, Aldoclor, Diupress

Actions
Diuretic; decreases reabsorption of chloride and sodium ions, which then leads to increased urinary output. Onset evident in 2 hours after oral ingestion.

Uses
Antihypertensive, diuretic, edema

Contraindications
Meds Hypersensitivity to sulfonamide-derived medications, lithium
Other Anuria, hepatic or renal dysfunction. *Use* with caution: Diabetes, gout, hypercalcemia, hyperuricemia, lupus erythematosus, pancreatitis, postsympathectomy

Interactions
Corticosteroids, corticotropin, oral antidiabetics

Dose
Adult PO: Antihypertensive: 500 mg bid; diuretic: 500 mg–1 gm qd–bid
Peds PO: 20 mg/kg/day in 2 divided doses

Forms
Oral suspension, sodium salt injection, syrup,
tablets

Adverse Effects
Anorexia, constipation, diarrhea, dizziness,
muscle cramps, nausea, orthostatic hypotension,
paresthesia, rash, urinary frequency, vomiting

**Special Nursing Considerations
and Patient Education**
- When used as a diuretic, administer in 1 dose in
  morning.
- Monitor blood pressure, I&O, weight.
- Give patient diet containing potassium-rich foods
  (see Appendix F).
- Discontinue for electrolyte imbalance.
- Be aware that
  – IV form is not recommended for children.
- Teach patient
  – that medication may cause photosensitivity.
  – to be cautious when driving or involved in
    potentially hazardous tasks.
  – to be cautious during hot weather or strenuous
    exercise because of hypotensive effects.
  – that urine output will increase.
  – techniques to avoid orthostatic hypotension
    (e.g., getting up slowly).
  – to decrease coffee, tea, and high-salt foods in
    diet.
  – to decrease smoking.
  – to take early in the day.

71

Chlorpheniramine Maleate/
Phenylephrine HCl/
Phenylpropanolamine HCl/
Phenyltoloxamine Citrate

Brand Name
Naldecon

Actions
Antihistamine, vasoconstrictor, vasopressor

Uses
Allergies, colds, orthostatic hypotension, upper
respiratory problems

Contraindications
Diabetes hypertension, hyperthyroidism, organic
cardiac disease

Interactions
None

Dose
Adult   1 tablet tid or 5 cc q3–4h
Peds   2.5–10 cc q3–4h

Forms
Pediatric syrup or drops, syrup, tablets

Adverse Effects
Anxiety, drowsiness, GI upset

**Special Nursing Considerations
and Patient Education**
- Administer after meals to decrease irritation.
- Teach patient
  - to be cautious when driving or involved in potentially hazardous tasks.

Chlorpromazine HCl

Brand Name
Thorazine

Actions
Antiemetic, antipsychotic, major tranquilizer.
Onset evident in 1–2 hours.

Uses
Acute intermittent porphyria, intractable
hiccoughs, nausea and vomiting, psychotic
disorders

Contraindications
Meds   Alcohol, CNS depressants
Other   Blood or bone-marrow disorders, children
under 6, coma. *Use with caution:* Cardiac,
hepatic, or respiratory dysfunction; epilepsy;
glaucoma; parkinsonism; peptic ulcer;
prostatic hypertrophy

Interactions
Antacids, antidiarrheals, atropine, guanethidine,
lithium, methyldopa, oral anticoagulants,
phenytoin, propranolol, trihexyphenidyl

Dose
Adult   PO: 25 mg–1 gm in divided doses
Peds   PO: 2 mg/kg/day in 4–6 divided doses

Forms
Capsules, injection, liquid, suppository, syrup,
tablets

Adverse Effects
Blood dycrasias, constipation, dry mouth,
extrapyramidal symptoms, hypothermia, jaundice,
orthostatic hypotension, sedation, urinary
retention, weight gain

**Special Nursing Considerations
and Patient Education**
• Store medication in light-resistant container.
• Inject IM dose deeply; maximum of 1 cc per site;
  massage injection site.
• When discontinued, decrease dosage gradually.
• Monitor blood pressure, fecal and urinary output,
  fluid intake.
• Monitor for fine vermicular tongue movements
  (may indicate early tardive dyskinesia).
• Offer hard candy (regular or sugar-free) to relieve
  dry mouth.
• Use caution when administering to a patient with
  suicidal potential; ensure patient swallows dose.
• Observe for extrapyramidal symptoms.
• Teach patient
    – to be cautious when driving or involved in
      potentially hazardous tasks.
    – to take precautions during hot weather or
      strenuous exercise because of hypotensive
      effects.
    – to notify physician for bleeding, impaired vision,
      jaundice, rash, sore throat, tremors, weakness.
    – to remain recumbent for ½ hour following
      parenteral dosage of medication.
    – that medication may color urine brown, pink, or
      red.
    – to change position slowly.
    – to use sunscreen.
    – to avoid alcohol, OTC medications.

Chlorpropamide

Brand Name
Diabinese

Actions
Antidiabetic, hypoglycemic; stimulates secretion of insulin from pancreas. Onset evident in 1 hour.

Uses
Diabetes (adult onset or noninsulin dependent)

Contraindications
Meds   Alcohol
Other   Diabetes associated with acidosis, infection, surgery, major trauma; endocrine, hepatic, or renal dysfunction; Insulin-dependent or juvenile diabetes. *Use with caution:* Peptic ulcer, porphyria, thyroid dysfunction

Interactions
Clofibrate, corticosteroids, digitoxin, insulin, MAO inhibitors, nonsteroidal anti-inflammatory agents, oral contraceptives, oxyphenbutazone, phenylbutazone, probenecid, salicylates, sulfonamides, thiazide diuretics

Dose
Adult   100–250 mg/day

Forms
Tablets

Adverse Effects
Diarrhea, GI problems, hepatic toxicities,
hypoglycemia, photosensitivity

**Special Nursing Considerations
and Patient Education**
- Monitor exercise, I&O, weight.
- Administer 30 minutes ac.
- Teach patient to
  - follow prescribed diet.
  - recognize signs of hyper- and hypoglycemia
    (see Appendix B).
  - take medication every day, except on
    professional advice.
  - avoid alcohol because of potential alcohol
    intolerance.
  - test urine glucose 1–3 x/day.
  - avoid OTC medications.
  - carry Medic-Alert ID.

Chlorzoxazone

Brand Name
Parafon Forte, Paraflex

Actions
Skeletal muscle relaxant; hinders multisynaptic
reflex arcs in subcortical brain and spinal cord.
Onset evident in 1 hour.

Uses
Adjunct in acute painful musculoskeletal
conditions

Contraindications
Alcohol, CNS depressants. *Use with caution:*
Hepatic or renal dysfunction, history of or known
allergies to muscle relaxants

Interactions
Antihistamines, barbiturates, hypnotics, sedatives,
tranquilizers

Dose
Adult   500–750 mg tid–qid
Peds   Based on age and weight: 125–500 mg tid-qid

Forms
Tablets

Adverse Effects

Angioneurotic edema, constipation, diarrhea,
dizziness, drowsiness, dyspepsia, ecchymosis,
headache, hepatic dysfunction, malaise, nausea,
petechiae, tarry stools, vertigo, vomiting

Special Nursing Considerations
and Patient Education

- Protect medication from light.
- Crush tablets tor easier administration.
- Assist with ambulation as necessary.
- Provide safety measures.
- Teach patient
  - that medication may color urine pink or red.
  - to be cautious when driving or involved in
    potentially hazardous tasks.
  - to avoid alcohol and other CNS depressants.
  - not to discontinue without physician's order.

Cholestyramine

Brand Name
Questran

Actions
Antilipemic; Increases oxidation of cholesterol into bile acids. Onset evident in 1 week.

Uses
Adjunct therapy in management of elevated cholesterol levels, pruritus caused by partial biliary obstruction

Contraindications
Complete biliary obstruction

Interactions
Digitalis, iron preparations, oral antibiotics or anticoagulants, phenylbutazone, thyroid hormones

Dose
Adult   4 gm tid–qid
Peds   Over 6 yr: 80 mg/kg tid

Forms
Powder

Adverse Effects

Anorexia; bleeding; bloating; constipation; diarrhea; fecal impaction; hyperchloremic acidosis; malabsorption of vitamins A,D,E,K; nausea

**Special Nursing Considerations
and Patient Education**

- Administer all other medications 1–4 hours before or after this medication.
- Teach patient
  - to follow prescribed diet and to include increased fluids and roughage.
  - that medication may cause burnt odor in urine and/or bad taste in mouth.
  - to use a stool softener to help ease constipation.
  - never take medication in dry form; mix slowly with liquids.
  - place powder on top of 4–6 ounces of liquid and twirl glass slowly for several minutes. After drinking the solution, refill glass with liquid and drink this also.
  - to report any dark, tarry stools, petechiae or hematuria to physician.

Cimetidine

Brand Name
Tagamet

Actions
Histamine antagonist. Onset of ulcer healing
evident in 2 weeks after initiation of therapy.

Uses
Duodenal or gastric ulcer, hypersecretory
disorders

Contraindications
Children under 16. *Use with caution:* Organic
brain syndrome, renal dysfunction

Actions
Antacids, coumarin anticoagulants, tricyclic
antidepressants

Dose
Adult   PO: 300 mg qid

Forms
Injection, liquid, tablets

Adverse Effects
Confusion, diarrhea, dizziness, gynecomastia,
headache, muscle pain, rash

**Special Nursing Considerations
and Patient Education**
- Administer IV over 2 30-minute period.
- Administer with meals.
- Administer antacids 1hour ac or 1 hour pc.
- Be aware that
  - treatment should only last for 8 weeks unless specifically directed otherwise by physician.
- Teach patient to
  - be cautious when driving or involved in potentially hazardous tasks.
  - follow dietary restrictions for ulcers.

Ciprofloxacin Hydrochloride

Brand Name
Cipro

Actions
Antibacterial. Onset evident in 1 hour.

Uses
Lower respiratory infection, skin and skin structure infections, bone and joint infections, urinary tract infections, infectious diarrhea

Contraindications
Hypersensitivity, radiation or/and chemotherapy within 1 month, thrombocytopenia, smallpox vaccination, CNS disorders

Interactions
Theophylline, magnesium hydroxide, aluminum hydroxide, probenecid

Dose
Adult   PO: UTI–mild/moderate: 250 mg q12h; UTI–complicated: 500 mg q12h; mild/moderate infection: 500 mg q12h; complicated infection: 750 mg q12h; infectious diarrhea: 500 mg q12h

Forms
Tablets

Adverse Effects
Nausea, diarrhea, vomiting, abdominal pain, headache, restlessness, rash, oral candidiasis, GI bleeding, pruritus, photosensitivity, fever, chills, blurred vision, tinnitus, dyspepsia, flatulence, confusion, increased BUN/SGOT/SGPT, decreased WBC

Special Nursing Considerations and Patient Education
- Administer 2 hours after meals.
- Encourage fluid intake to 3 liters/day.
- Assess CNS symptoms.
- Obtain urines for culture and sensitivity.
- Administer with food or milk to decrease GI discomfort.
- Teach patient to
  - not take antacid with magnesium or aluminum while on this medication.
  - use sunscreen.
  - take full prescription.

Clemastine Fumarate USP

Brand Name
Tavist-D

Actions
Antihistamine, nasal decongestant. Peak
response in 4 hours.

Uses
Relief of allergy symptoms—sneezing, rhinorrhea,
pruritus, lacrimation, nasal congestion

Contraindications
Hypersensitivity to components, asthma, severe
hypertension, severe coronary artery disease.
Use with caution: narrow-angle glaucoma,
stenosing peptic ulcer, pyloroduodenal
obstruction, sympathomatic prostatic hypertrophy,
bladder-neck obstruction, hypertension,
cardiovascular disease, diabetes mellitus,
uncontrolled hyperthyroidism

Interactions
MAO inhibitors, alcohol, CNS depressants,
methyldopa, mecamylamine, reserpine

Dose
Adult   PO: 1 tablet q12h

Forms
Tablets

Adverse Effects
Sedation, dizziness, disturbed coordination, epigastric distress, thickening of bronchial secretions, rash dryness of mouth/nose/throat, headache, urinary retention, hypertension, constipation, hypotension

Special Nursing Considerations and Patient Education
- Offer hard, sugar-free candy to relieve dry mouth.
- Assess I&O.
- Administer with food.
- Teach patient to
  - not take alcohol or OTC medications.
  - not drive while taking medication.
  - change position slowly.

Clindamycin Hydrochloride

Brand Name

Cleocin

Actions

Lincosamide antibiotic. Onset evident: rapid.

Uses

Serious infection caused by susceptible strains of anaerobes, streptocci, staphylocci, pneumocci, adjunct to surgical treatment of chronic bone and joint infections, treatment of acne vulgaris (topical)

Contraindications

Hypersensitivity to clindamycin or lincomycin. *Use with caution:* history of gastrointestinal disease, colitis, atopic individuals, renal and liver disease

Interactions

Chloramphenicol, erythromycin, nondepolarizing muscle relaxants, Kaolin

Dose

Adult   PO: 150–450 mg q6h; IM/IV: 300 mg q6–12h; *maximum* dose: 4800 mg/day

Peds   PO: 8–25 mg/kg/day in divided doses q6–8h; IM/IV: 15–40 mg/kg/day in divided doses q6–8h

Forms
Capsules, injection

Adverse Effects
Abdominal pain, nausea, vomiting, diarrhea,
vaginitis, headache, dizziness, jaundice, rash,
abcess at injection site

**Special Nursing Considerations
and Patient Education**
- Administer IV by infusion only.
- Reconstitute by adding 75 ml water to 100 ml
  bottle; shake well; do not refrigerate.
- Administer IM dose with deep injection; rotate
  sites.
- Do not administer IM greater than 600 mg.
- Assess bowel patterns.
- Administer with food to decrease GI discomfort.
- Assess blood studies, liver studies.
- Teach patient to
  - discontinue if diarrhea occurs.
  - take PO with a full glass of water.
  - notify physician if fever, fatigue or sore throat
    occur.
  - take medication around the clock at equal
    intervals.

Clonazepam

Brand Name
Clonopin, Klonopin, Rivotril

Actions
Anticonvulsant; affects minor motor seizures (amplitude, duration, frequency, spread of discharge). Onset evident: 20–60 minutes.

Uses
Akinesia, Lennox-Gastat syndrome, myoclonic seizures

Contraindications
Meds Alcohol, antihistamines, barbiturates, CNS depressants, hypnotics, narcotics, phenothiazines, sedatives, tricyclic antidepressants
Other Acute narrow-angle glaucoma, hepatic dysfunction

Interactions
Phenobarbital, phenytoin, CNS depressants

Dose
Adult Initial Dose: 1.5 mg/day In 3 divided doses; dosage may be increased in increments of 0.5–1 mg q3days until seizures are controlled; *maximum* dose: 20 mg/day
Peds Up to 10 yr: 0.01–0.03 mg/kg/day in 2–3 divided dose; over 10 yr: same as adult

Forms
  Tablets

Adverse Effects
  Anemia, anorexia, aphonia, ataxia, behavior
  problems, bruising, chest congestion, choreiform
  movements, confusion, depression, drowsiness,
  dry mouth, encopresis, hallucinations, palpitations,
  psychoses, rhinorrhea

**Special Nursing Considerations
and Patient Education**
- Use caution when administering to patients with
  suicidal potential, ensure patient swallows dose.
- Monitor seizure activity.
- Offer hard candy (regular or sugar-free) to relieve
  dry mouth.
- May crush tablets.
- Institute seizure precautions.
- May administer with food.
- Be aware that
  - medication can cause dependence; when
    discontinued, decrease dosage gradually.
- Teach patient
  - to be cautious when driving or involved in
    potentially hazardous tasks.
  - that medication may cause an increase in
    salivation or a feeling of coated tongue.
  - to carry some type of Medic Alert card or
    bracelet.
  - avoid alcohol, OTC medications.

Clonidine HCl

Brand Name
Catapres, Combipres

Actions
Vasodilator; decreases ability of sympathetic nervous system to maintain blood vessel constriction. Onset evident in 30–60 minutes.

Uses
Antihypertensive, withdrawal from narcotics (investigational use)

Contraindications
Meds Alcohol, CNS depressants
Other Children, diabetes. *Use with caution:* Cardiovascular dysfunction, chronic renal failure

Interactions
Tolazoline, tricyclic antidepressants

Dose
Adult Initial dose: 0.1 mg bid; maximum effective dose: 2.4 mg/day

Forms
Tablets, transdermal patch

Adverse Effects
Bradycardia, congestive heart failure, constipation, depression, drowsiness, dry mouth,

fatigue, headache, insomnia, nausea, orthostatic hypotension, vivid dreams, vomiting, weight gain

Special Nursing Considerations and Patient Education

- Take blood pressure prior to administering medication and during treatment.
- Monitor behavioral changes, blood pressure, I&O, neurologic status, weight.
- When discontinued, decrease dosage gradually over 2–4 days; give last dose at hs.
- Offer hard candy (regular or sugar-free) to relieve dry mouth.
- Apply transdermal patch every 7 days.
- Be aware that
  - tolerance can develop.
  - if discontinued abruptly, a rapid increase in blood pressure is possible.
- Teach patient
  - to be cautious when driving or involved in potentially hazardous tasks.
  - about the possibility of weight gain and individually prescribed weight-control diet.
  - to monitor blood pressure for a month following discontinuation of treatment.
  - to change position slowly to avoid orthostatic hypotension.

Clorazepate Dipotassium

Brand Name
Tranxene

Actions
Depresses subcortical levels of CNS. Onset evident in 30–60 minutes.

Uses
Anxiety disorders, short-term relief of anxiety symptoms, adjunctive therapy in management of partial seizures, relief of acute alcohol withdrawal symptoms

Contraindications
Depressive neurosis, psychotic reactions, acute narrow-angle glaucoma. *Use with caution:* suicidal tendencies, impaired renal or hepatic function, elderly or debilitated patients

Interactions
Oral contraceptives, valproic acid, CNS depressants, alcohol, disulfiram, antihistamines, narcotics, hypnotics.

Dose
Adult PO: anxiety: 15–60 mg/day in divided doses; alcohol withdrawal: day 1: 30 mg, then 30–60 mg/day; day 2: 45–90 mg in divided doses; day 3: 22.5–45 mg in divided doses;

94

day 4: 15–30 mg in divided doses; reduce
daily to 7.5–15 mg; seizure: 7.5 mg tid; may
increase 7.5 mg/week; *maximum* dose: 90
mg/day
Peds   PO: seizure: 7.5 mg bid; may increase 7.5
mg/week; *maximum* dose: 60 mg/day

Forms
  Tablets

Adverse Effects
  Drowsiness, dizziness, GI discomfort,
  nervousness, dry mouth, mental confusion,
  orthostatic hypotension, blurred vision, lethargy,
  psychological or physical dependence.

**Special Nursing Considerations
and Patient Education**
• Monitor seizure activity, level of anxiety.
• Administer with food to decrease GI discomfort.
• Offer hard, sugar-free candy to relieve dry mouth.
• Be sure patient swallows the medication.
• Teach patient to
  – change position slowly.
  – take only as prescribed.
  – avoid alcohol.
  – notify physician if preganancy is suspected.
  – avoid OTC counter medications.

Clotrimazole

Brand Name
Lotrimin, Gyne-Lotrimin, Mycelex, Myclex-G

Actions
Antifungal—broad spectrum. Onset evident: PO
15–30 minutes. Topical and vaginal upon
application.

Uses
Treatment of tinea pedis, tinea cruris and tinea
corporis due to trichophyton rubrum, trichophyton
mentagropheytes, Epidermophyton floccosum
and Microsporum canis; treatment of candidiasis
due to Candida albicans; treatment of tinea
versicolor due to Malassezia furfur

Contraindications
Hypersensitivity

Interactions
None

Dose
Adult & Peds   PO: 10 mg lozenge dissolved slowly
5 ×/day; topical: apply bid to affected area;
vaginal tablets: 100 mg vaginally × 7 days,
or 200 mg qd × 3 days, or 5 g of vaginal
cream qd × 7–14 days

**Special Nursing Considerations
and Patient Education**
- Assess affect skin areas frequently for irritation.
- Do not apply to areas surrounding eyes.
- Provide good hygiene.
- Teach patient to
  - let lozenge dissolve; do not swallow or chew.
  - apply cream with gloves.
  - apply vaginal creams and tablets properly; lie down for 10–15 minutes after application.
  - wear sanitary pad to prevent staining.
  - use full course of treatment.
  - notify physician if signs of increased irritation occur.
  - continue during menstrual cycle.
  - refrain from sexual intercourse or partner should wear condom.

Codeine Phosphate, Sulfate

Brand Name
Methylmorphine

Actions
Narcotic; acts on CNS and GI tract. Onset evident in 15–30 minutes.

Uses
Analgesic, antitussive

Contraindications
Meds Alcohol, hypersensitivity to narcotics, MAO inhibitors
Other Bronchial asthma, head injuries, respiratory depression. *Use with caution:* Addison's disease, cardiac dysrhythmias, chronic ulcerative colitis, gallbladder, hepatic or renal dysfunction, prostatic hypertrophy, urethral stricture

Interactions
Anticholinergics, antidepressants, antihistamines, general anesthetics, hypnotics, MAO inhibitors, phenothiazines, sedatives, skeletal muscle relaxants, tranquilizers, tricyclic antidepressants

Dose
Adult PO: Analgesic: 15–60 mg qid; antitussive: 8–20 mg q3–4h

Peds PO: Analgesic: 3 mg/kg/day in 6 divided
doses; antitussive: 1–1.5 mg/day in 6 divided
doses

Forms
Phosphate injection, syrup, tablets

Adverse Effects
Constipation, dizziness, drowsiness, excitement,
restlessness

**Special Nursing Considerations
and Patient Education**
- Store medication in light-resistant container.
- When discontinued, decrease dosage gradually.
- Be aware that
  - usual preparations are combinations of 2 or
    more drugs.
  - medication can be habit forming.
- Teach patient
  - to be cautious when driving or involved in
    potentially hazardous tasks.

Co-Trimoxazole

Brand Name
Bactrim, Cotrim, Comoxol, Septra, Sulfatrim,
Bethaprim

Actions
Antibiotic. Onset evident: rapid.

Uses
Urinary tract infection, acute otitis media, acute
bronchitis, shigellosis, pneumocystis, carinii
pneumonia

Contraindications
Hypersensitivity, megaloblastic anemia,
streptoccal pharyngitis, pregnancy at term,
acquired immunodeficiency syndrome. *Use with
caution*: impaired renal function

Interactions
Phenytoin, oral hypoglycemics, oral
anticoagulants, methotrexate, thiazides

Dose
Adult   PO: UTI, Shifellosis, acute otitis media: 160
mg Trimethoprim/800 mg Sulfamethoxazole
q12h; chronic bronchitis: 160 mg
Trimethoprim/800 mg Sulfamethoxazole
q12h; pneumocystis carinii pneumonia: PO/

IV: 5mg/kg Trimethoprim/25mg
Sulfamethoxazole q6h

Peds PO: UTI, Shifellosis, acute otitis media: 7.5–
8 mg/kg Trimethoprim/37.5–40 mg/kg
Sulfamethoxazole qd in divided doses q12h;
pneumocystis carinii pneumonia: PO/IV:
5mg/kg Trimethoprim/25mg
Sulfamethoxazole q6h

Forms
Tablets, IV solution, liquid

Adverse Effects
Rash, nausea, vomiting, headache, insomnia,
depression, fatigue, abdominal pain, anxiety,
anorexia, urticaria, photosensitivity

Special Nursing Considerations
and Patient Education
- Provide increased fluids.
- Monitor C & S prior to and during treatment.
- Monitor I&O.
- Administer 1 hour ac or 1 hour pc with water.
- IV—dilute 5 ml ampule with 125 ml D5W.
- Do not refrigerate IV solution.
- Use IV immediately after reconstituting.
- Teach patient to
  - increase fluid intake.
  - take medication around the clock.
  - use sunscreen.
  - notify physician if rash, sore throat or fever
    occur.
  - take with a full glass of water.
  - take full prescribed amount.   101
  - use alternative contraceptive measures.

Cromolyn Sodium

Brand Name
Intal, Nasalcrom

Actions
Antiasthmatic, antihistamine. Onset evident:
Inhalation—within 2–4; weeks; nasal—less than 1
week.

Uses
Prevention and treatment of allergic rhinitis
symptoms, severe bronchial asthma, prevention
of exercise-induced bronchospasm

Contraindications
Hypersensitivity

Interactions
None

Dose
Adult & Peds   (over 6 yr.) 1 spray/nostril tid–qid;
    may increase up to 6 ×/day

Forms
Metered spray bottle

Adverse Effects
Sneezing, nasal stinging, nasal burning, nasal
irritation, headaches, bad taste

**Special Nursing Considerations
and Patient Education**
- Assess pulmonary function, lung sounds prior to and during treatment.
- Inform patient that therapeutic effects may take up to 4 weeks.
- Teach patient to
    - use inhaler properly.
    - gargle after treatments.
    - clear mucous prior to treatment.

Cyclobenzaprine HCl

Brand Name
Flexeril

Actions
Central-acting muscle relaxant. Onset evident in 1 hour.

Uses
Adjunct in acute, painful musculoskeletal conditions

Contraindications
Meds Alcohol, CNS depressants, MAO inhibitors
Other Cardiac dysrhythmias, children under 15, congestive heart failure, heart block, hyperthyroidism, recovering MI. *Use with caution:* History of urinary retention

Interactions
Anticholinergics, guanethidine

Dose
Adult 10 mg tid; not recommended for use longer than 2–3 weeks

Forms
Tablets

Adverse Effects
Blurred vision, cardiac irregularities, dizziness, drowsiness, dry mouth, dyspepsia, insomnia, paresthesia, tachycardia, weakness

**Special Nursing Considerations
and Patient Education**
- Administer for 2–3 weeks only.
- When discontinued, decrease dosage gradually.
- Offer hard candy (regular or sugar-free) to relieve dry mouth.
- Teach patient to
  – be cautious when driving or involved in potentially hazardous tasks.

Demeclocycline HCl

Brand Name
Declomycin

Actions
Antiamebic, antibacterial, antibiotic, anti-infective, antirickettsial; hinders protein synthesis in select microorganisms. Onset evident in 2–5 days.

Uses
Granuloma inguinale, lymphogranuloma, mycoplasms, ornithosis, psittacosis, rickettsial disease, spirochetal relapsing fever

Contraindications
Meds　Antacids, antidiarrheals, dairy products
Other　Children under 9, renal dysfunction. *Use with caution:* Hepatic or renal dysfunction

Interactions
Anticoagulants, iron and mineral preparations, methoxyflurane, sodium bicarbonate

Dose
Adult　150 mg q6h or 300 mg q12h
Peds　Over 9 yr: 3–6 mg/kg/day in 2–4 divided doses

Forms
Capsules, tablets

Adverse Effects
Diabetes insipidus syndrome, increased skin pigmentation, nausea, superinfections

**Special Nursing Considerations
and Patient Education**
- Store in light-resistant containers.
- Administer oral forms 1 hour before or 2 hours after meals.
- Monitor I&O if therapy is prolonged.
- Teach patient
  - that medication may cause photosensitivity.
  - to take entire course of treatment.
  - to avoid milk products.

Desipramine HCl

Brand Name
Norpramin, Pertofrane

Actions
Antidepressant. Onset evident in 1–2 weeks.

Uses
Endogenous or reactive depression

Contraindications
Meds Alcohol, MAO Inhibitors
Other Children, narrow-angle glaucoma, recent MI.
Use with caution: Asthma, cardiac disease, diabetes, epilepsy, hyperthyroid, bipolar disorders, prostatic hypertrophy, psychoses

Interactions
Adrenergics, anticholinergics, antihistamines, clonidine, ethchlorvynol, guanethidine, hypnotics, narcotics, procainamide, quinidine, sedatives, thyroid preparations, tranquilizers

Dose
Adult 25–50 mg tid; dosage above 300 mg/day not recommended
Peds Adolescent: 25–100 mg/day

Forms
Capsules, tablets

Adverse Effects
Blurred vision, constipation, dizziness,
drowsiness, dry mouth, impaired urination

Special Nursing Considerations
and Patient Education
- Use caution when administering to a patient with
  suicidal potential; ensure patient swallows dose.
- Monitor blood pressure until dosage is regulated.
- Administer with food to decrease GI discomfort.
- Offer hard candy (regular or sugar-free) to relieve
  dry mouth.
- When discontinued, decrease dosage gradually.
- Teach patient
  - to change position slowly to avoid orthostatic
    hypotension.
  - that medication may cause photosensitivity and
    peculiar taste in mouth.
  - to be cautious when driving or involved in
    potentially hazardous tasks.
  - to refrain from taking other medications for 2
    weeks following discontinuation of this
    medication.

Desoximetasone

Brand Name
Topicort, Topicort LP

Actions
Topical corticosteroid

Uses
Inflammatory and pruritic manifestations of
dermatoses: psoriasis, eczema, pruritis, contact
dermatitis

Contraindications
Hypersensitivity

Interactions
None

Dose
Adult   Apply thin coat to affected area bid

Forms
Topical cream

Adverse Effects
Burning, itching, irritation, dryness, folliculitis,
hypertrichosis, hypopigmentation, perioral
dermatitis, secondary infection

110

**Special Nursing Considerations
and Patient Education**
- Do not cover affected area.
- Cleanse area prior to application.
- Teach patient to
  - properly apply medication.

Desoxyribonuclease/Fibrinolysin

Brand Name
Elase

Actions
Topical enzyme

Uses
Circumcision, episiotomy, 2nd and 3rd degree burns, surgical wounds, ulcerative lesions

Contraindications
Hypersensitivity. *Use with caution:* Sensitivity to bovine origin materials

Interactions
None

Dose
Adult   Apply bid–tid q6–10h
Peds   Same as adult

Forms
Ointment, powder (for solution)

Adverse Effects
Angioneurotic edema, maculopapular or vesicular dermatitis, pruritus, urticaria

**Special Nursing Considerations
and Patient Education**
- Refrigerate ointment.
- Do not use reconstituted solutions after 24 hours.
- Monitor condition of wound.
- Use aseptic technique with wounds.

Dexamethasone

Brand Name
Decadron, Dexone, Hexadrol

Actions
Anti-inflammatory, glucocorticoid. Onset evident in 24–48 hours.

Uses
Allergies, cerebral edema resulting from brain metastasis, inflammations

Contraindications
Active eye infection, peptic ulcer, or tuberculosis; systemic fungal infection. *Use with caution:* Diabetes, glaucoma, hypertension, hypothyroidism, myasthenia gravis, thrombophlebitis

Interactions
Barbiturates, coumarin anticoagulants, digitalis preparations, ephedrine, insulin, oral antidiabetics, phenytoin, rifampin

Dose
Adult   PO: 0.5–9 mg/day
Peds   PO: 0.2 mg/kg/day in divided doses

Forms
Aerosol inhaler or skin spray, elixir, cream, injection, liquid, ophthalmic ointment or solution, tablets

Adverse Effects
Dry nose, epistaxis, fluid and electrolyte
disturbances, headache, hypertension, insomnia,
retention of sodium

**Special Nursing Considerations
and Patient Education**
- Monitor height (children), weight.
- Give high-protein diet.
- Monitor I&O, weight.
- Administer with meals.
- Be aware that
  - medication may cause dependence; when
    discontinued, decrease dosage gradually.
- Teach patient to
  - stop/decrease smoking.
  - carry some type of Medic Alert card or bracelet.
  - notify physician of menstrual irregularities,
    muscle weakness, vertigo.
  - (diabetic patient) test urine for glucose at least
    daily.
  - avoid possible infections.

Dextroamphetamine Sulfate

Brand Name
Dexedrine

Actions
Anorexiant, cerebral stimulant, sympathomimetic.
Onset evident in 30–60 minutes.

Uses
Adjunct in treatment of obesity, minimal brain
dysfunction, narcolepsy

Contraindications
Meds MAO inhibitors
Other Agitated states, angina pectoris,
arteriosclerosis, cardiovascular disease,
diabetes, history of drug abuse,
hyperexcitability, hypertension,
hyperthyroidism, nephritis, tension. *Use with
caution:* Arteriosclerosis, CVA, glaucoma;
hypertension, psychoses

Interactions
Antihypertensives, insulin, tricyclic
antidepressants

Dose
Adult 2.5–10 mg qd–tid; narcolepsy: 5–60 mg/day
Peds 2–15 mg/day in 2–3 divided doses

116

Forms
Elxir, long-acting capsules, tablets

Adverse Effects
Anorexia, constipation, diarrhea, dizziness, dry mouth, insomnia, nausea, nervousness, restlessness

Special Nursing Considerations and Patient Education
- Do not crush long-acting capsules.
- Monitor vital signs daily.
- Do not administer Within 6 hours of hs.
- Offer hard candy (regular or sugar-free) to relieve dry mouth.
- Be aware that
  - medication may be habit forming; when discontinued, decrease dosage gradually.
- Teach patient
  - that medication may cause a metallic taste in mouth.
  - to avoid foods rich in tyramine (see Appendix F).
  - to be cautious when driving or involved in potentially hazardous tasks.
  - if hypertensive, to use caution during strenuous activities and to recognize signs of hypertensive difficulty (e.g., easy fatigue, headache, irritability, nervousness).

Dextromethorphan Hydrobromide with Iodinated Glycerol

Brand Name
Tussi-Organiden

Actions
Antitussive mucolytic expectorant

Uses
Irritating non-productive cough associated with chronic bronchitis, bronchial asthma, common cold; symptomatic relief of cough associated with laryngitis, pharyngitis, croup, pertussis, emphysema

Contraindications
Hypersensitivity. *Use with caution:* cystic fibrosis, thyroid disease

Interactions
Lithium, anti-thyroid medications.

Dose
Adult   PO: 1–2 tsp. q4h
Peds   PO: ½–1 tsp q4h

Forms
Liquid

118

Adverse Effects

Rash, GI irritation, nausea, vomiting, constipation, drowsiness, thyroid gland enlargement

Special Nursing Considerations
and Patient Education

- Inform patient that medication may be habit forming.
- Administer with food to decrease GI discomfort.
- Teach patient to
  - follow physician's orders for primary disease.
  - notify physician of suspected pregnancy, rash.
  - avoid driving, alcohol, OTC medications.

Diazepam

Brand Name
Valium

Actions
Amnesic, anticonvulsant, hypnotic, sedative, skeletal muscle relaxant; depresses brainstem reticular formation and limbic system. Onset evident: PO 30–60 minutes; IM 15–30 minutes.

Uses
Anxiety, diagnostic tests (e.g., cardioversion, esophagoscopy, gastroscopy), muscle spasms, preoperative, status epilepticus, tension, withdrawal from alcohol

Contraindications
Meds Alcohol, MAO inhibitors
Other Acute alcohol intoxication, children (IM/IV: under 1 month; PO: under 6 months), coma, myasthenia gravis, narrow-angle glaucoma, shock. *Use with caution:* Depression; hepatic, pulmonary, or renal dysfunction; psychoses

Interactions
Anticonvulsants, antidepressants, CNS depressants, hypnotics, narcotics, sedatives, tranquilizers

Dose

Adult PO: 2–10 mg bid–qid
Peds PO: Over 6 months: 1–2.5 mg tid–qid
Over 1 month: 1–2 mg q3–4h IM/IV

Forms
Injection, tablets

Adverse Effects
Dizziness, drowsiness, headache, hypotension,
libido changes, nausea

**Special Nursing Considerations
and Patient Education**
- Do not allow IV to exceed 5 mg/minute.
Use caution when administering to a patient with
suicidal potential; ensure patient swallows dose.
- Discontinue for bruising, eye pain, fever,
hemorrhage, sore throat.
- Be aware that
  - IM Dose is absorbed erratically and painfully.
  - medication is cumulative and causes
dependence; when discontinued, decrease
dosage gradually.
  - medication may increase possibility of
convulsions.

Diclofenac

Brand Name
Voltaren

Actions
Anti-inflammatory (non-steroid)

Uses
Acute and chronic rheumatoid arthritis,
osteoarthristis and ankylosing spondylitis

Contraindications
Hypersentivity to the medication, aspirin and other
non-steroidals, anti-inflammatory medications.
Use with caution: GI disorders, cardiac disorders

Interactions
Aspirin, anticoagulants, digoxin, methotrexate,
cyclosporine, lithium, diuretics, probenecid, beta-
blockers

Dose
Adult: PO: osteoarthritis: 100–150 mg/day in
divided doses; rheumatoid arthritis: 150–200
mg/day in divided doses; ankylosing
spondylitis 100–125 mg/day qid, hs

Forms
Tablets—coated

Adverse Effects
Nausea and vomiting, constipation, GI bleeding, dizziness, confusion, headache, abdominal pain, diarrhea, fluid retention, rash, tinnitus

Special Nursing Considerations and Patient Education
- Monitor blood count during therapy.
- Observe for signs and symptoms of G1 bleeding.
- Administer with food and/or milk.
- Teach the patient to
    - report signs of bleeding, bruising to physician.
    - avoid aspirin.
    - take with milk and/or food.

Diflunisal

Brand Name
Dolobid

Actions
Non-narcotic analgesic, anti-inflammatory, nonsteroidal anti-inflammatory, antipyretic. Onset evident in 60 minutes.

Uses
Mild to moderate pain, osteoarthritis, rheumatoid arthritis

Contraindications
Hypersensitivity to salicylates, GI bleeding. *Use with caution*: renal or hepatic dysfunction, history of ulcers, bleeding disorders

Interactions
Anticoagulants, hydrochlorothiazide, antacids, steroids, acetaminophen, probenecid, salicylates

Dose
Adult PO: pain initial dose: 500–1000 mg, then 250–500 mg q8–12h; inflammatory: 500–1000 mg/ day in divided doses; *maximum* dose: 1500 mg/day

Forms
   Tablets

Adverse Effects
   Nausea, vomiting, GI pain, diarrhea, flatulence,
   constipation, insomnia, dizziness, rash, headache,
   tinnitus, fatigue, heartburn, GI bleeding

**Special Nursing Considerations
and Patient Education**
- Administer with food or milk to decrease GI
  discomfort.
- Monitor blood studies if on long-term therapy.
- Monitor I&O.
- Administer tablet whole; do not crush.
- Provide comfort measures concurrently.
- Teach patient to
    - take as prescribed.
    - avoid OTC medications containing aspirin.
    - avoid alcohol.
    - report signs of GI bleeding immediately.
    - take with 8 ounces of fluid and remain upright
      for 30 minutes.

Digitoxin

Brand Name
Crystodigin, Purodigin, Unidigin

Actions
Cardiac glycoside; increases availability of calcium in heart muscle. Onset evident: PO 2–4 hours; IV 30 minutes–2 hours.

Uses
Dysrhythmias

Contraindications
Hepatic damage. *Use with caution:* Cardiac block, emphysema, hepatic or renal dysfunction, hypercalcemia, hypertrophic subaortic stenosis, hypokalemia, hypothyroidism, MI, myocarditis, myxedema, ventricular fibrillation

Interactions
Adrenergic agents, calcium. procainamide, propranolol, quinidine, thyroid preparations

Dose
Adult　PO: Digitalizing dose 1.2–1.6 mg; *maintenance* dose 0.05–0.3 mg/day

Peds　PO: 1 month–2 yr: *digitalizing* dose 0.04 mg/kg;
over 2 yr: *digitalizing* dose 0.03 mg/kg; *maintenance dose:* 1/10 of digitalizing dose

Forms
   Injection, tablets

Adverse Effects
   Anorexia, confusion, diarrhea, disorientation,
   drowsiness, headache, increased salivation,
   irregular pulse, irritability, nausea, restlessness,
   visual disturbances, vomiting

Special Nursing Considerations
and Patient Education
* Take apical pulse prior to administration; if a
  change is noted, hold dose until you confer with
  physician. Monitor pulse as necessary per
  individual patient.
* Give IM dose deep into gluteal muscle, no more
  than 2 cc/site; massage site after injection.
* Notify physician of anorexia, dysrhythmias,
  blurred vision, diarrhea, irregular pulse, nausea,
  visual color disturbances.
* Protect medication from light.
* Be aware that
  – maintenance dose is usually given as a single
    dose in morning with meal.
* Teach patient
  – to decrease caffeine intake and smoking
    because of their stimulant effect.
  – of the possibility of taking medication for a
    lifetime.

Digoxin

Brand Name
Lanoxin

Actions
Cardiotonic digitalis glycoside; increases force of myocardial contractions

Uses
Atrial fibrillation and flutter, congestive heart failure, paroxysmal atrial tachycardia

Contraindications
Complete atrio-ventricular block, ventricular tachycardia. *Use with caution:* Acute MI, emphysema, glomerulonephritis, hypercalcemia, idiopathic hypertrophic subaortic stenosis, ischemic cardiac or renal dysfunction, myocarditis, myxedema, pericarditis, increased serum potassium, rheumatic carditis, ventricular fibrillation

Interactions
Adrenergic agents, calcium, procainamide, propranolol, quinidine, thyroid preparations

Dose
Adult Digitalization; initial dose, PO: 2–3 mg; IV: 1–1.5 mg; IM: 1–2 mg; *maintenance* dose: 0.125–0.50 mg/day PO

Peds Digitalization; newborn: initial dose, 0.04–0.06 mg/kg PO; 1 month–2 yr: 0.06–0.08 mg/kg; over 2 yrs: 0.04–0.06 mg/kg; *maintenance dose:* usually 1/5–1/3 of
128   digitalizing dose

Forms
Elixir, injection, pediatric elixir and injection, tablets

Adverse Effects
Anorexia, diarrhea, drowsiness, fatigue, increased salivation, irregular pulse, nausea, pedal edema, vomiting, weakness; *in neonates:* prolongation of P-R interval, sinoatrial arrest, undue slowing of sinus rate

Special Nursing Considerations and Patient Education
- Take apical/radial pulse for 1 minute prior to administration. Hold drug if rate is less than 60 for adults, 70 for pediatric patients. Identify individualized pulse monitoring guidelines.
- Inject IM dose into deep muscles; give no more than 2 cc at 1 site; massage site after administration.
- Protect medication from light.
- Monitor I&0; take weight daily.
- Be aware that
  - therapy with this medication is usually ongoing.
- Teach patient to
  - carry some type of Medic Alert card or bracelet.
  - notify physician of anorexia, dysrhythmias, blurred vision, changes in pulse rate or regularity, diarrhea, nausea, visual color disturbances.
  - take at the same time each day.

Diltiazem Hydrochloride

Brand Name
Cardizem

Actions
Coronary vasodilator, calcium channel blocker, antianginal, antihypertensive. Onset evident in 30–60 minutes.

Uses
Chronic stable angina pectoris, coronary artery spasm, hypertension, Prinzmetal's variant angina

Contraindications
Sick sinus syndrome (without a pacemaker), second or third degree AV block (without a pacemaker), hypotension, hypersensitivity, acute myocardial infarction and pulmonary congestion, acute hepatic injury

Interactions
Beta-adrenergic blockers, digoxin, lithium, cimetidine, anesthetics

Dose
Adult   PO: 30 mg qid; increase to 240 mg/day in divided doses

Forms
Tablets

Adverse Effects
Arrhythmias, constipation, edema, fatigue, headache, hypotension, rash

Special Nursing Considerations and Patient Education
- Assess for signs of congestive heart failure.
- Monitor for signs and symptoms of digitalis toxicity if patient is receiving digoxin concurrently.
- Monitor I&O.
- Monitor vital signs prior to administration.
- Provide small, frequent meals if nausea or GI problems occur.
- Teach patient
  - take pulse prior to administration.
  - change positions slowly because of orthostatic hypotension.
  - use sunscreen to avoid photosensitive reaction.
  - contact physician if chest pain increases or shortness of breath occurs.
  - avoid OTC drugs unless physician approves.

Dimenhydrinate

Brand Name
Dramamine

Actions
Antinauseant; decreases motion-caused stimulation of labyrinth structures. Onset evident in 30–60 minutes.

Uses
Dizziness, nausea, vertigo, vomiting associated with motion sickness

Contraindications
Meds Alcohol, CNS depressants, MAO inhibitors, ototoxics
Other Allergies to diphenhydramine or theophylline; infants, neonates. *Use with caution:* Bladder-neck or pyloroduodenal obstruction, cardiovascular dysfunction, history of reactions to antihistamines, hypertension, hyperthyroidism, narrow-angle glaucoma, prostatic hypertrophy, stenosing peptic ulcer

Interactions
Aminoglycosides, tricyclic antidepressants

Dose
Adult PO: 50–100 mg q4h; parenteral: 50 mg prn
Peds PO: Over 3 yr: 1.25 mg/kg qid

132

Forms
Injection, suppository, syrup, tablets

Adverse Effects
Blurred vision, dizziness, drowsiness, headache, nausea, palpitations

Special Nursing Considerations and Patient Education
- Be aware that tolerance can develop.
- Administer 30 minutes prior to travel to prevent motion sickness; preferably 1–2 hours prior to travel.
- Teach patient to
  - be cautious when driving or involved in potentially hazardous tasks.
  - avoid alcohol.

Diphenhydramine HCl

Brand Name
Benadryl, Benylin

Actions
Antiemetic, antiparkinsonism, antivertigo, histamine antagonist, hypnotic. Onset evident in 30 minutes.

Uses
Allergic reactions (blood, blood plasma, conjunctivitis, rhinitis), angioedema, intractable insomnia, motion sickness, parkinsonism, pruritus, urticaria

Contraindications

Meds Alcohol, CNS depressants, MAO inhibitors

Other Acute asthma, lactation, narrow-angle glaucoma, urinary retention. *Use with caution:* Cardiovascular disease, hypertension, hyperthyroidism, prostatic hypertrophy, pyloroduodenal obstruction, stenosing peptic ulcer

Interactions
Epinephrine, phenothiazines

Dose

Adult PO: 25–50 mg tid–qld

Peds PO: 5 mg/kg in 4 divided doses

Forms
   Capsules, elixir, injection

Adverse Effects
   Constipation, dizziness, drowsiness, epigastric
   distress, headache, hypotension, nausea,
   tachycardia, vomiting

**Special Nursing Considerations
and Patient Education**
- Administer IV dose slowly, with patient recumbent.
- Counsel patient to avoid alcohol.
- Monitor impact of medication on the blood
  pressure of patients with blood pressure
  dysfunction.
- Give drug with meals or milk to reduce GI upset.
- Protect medication from light.
- Teach patient
  - to be cautious when driving or involved in
    potentially hazardous tasks.
  - that medication may cause decreased tolerance
    to contact lenses because of atropine-like
    effects.

Diphenoxylate HCl/ Atropine Sulfate

Brand Name
Lomotil

Actions
Antidiarrheal; slows intestinal motility. Onset evident in 45–60 minutes.

Uses
Colostomy, diarrhea, ileostomy

Contraindications
Meds MAO inhibitors
Other Children under 2, cirrhosis, colitis, diarrhea as a result of poisoning, glaucoma, hepatic disease, jaundice. *Use with caution:* Addison's disease, cardiovascular instability, dehydration, diarrhea (infection), gallbladder or hepatic disease, hiatal hernia, hypertension, hyperthyroidism, hypothyroidism, intestinal atony, myasthenia gravis, prostatic hypertrophy, renal dysfunction, urethral stricture

Interactions
Alcohol, amantadine, atropine-like drugs, barbiturates, CNS depressants, haloperidol, hypnotics, narcotics, phenothiazines, sedatives, tranquilizers, tricyclic antidepressants

Dose

Adult 5 mg tid–qid
Peds 2–12 yr: (liquid only) 0.3–0.4 mg/kg/day in
divided doses

Forms
Liquid, tablets

Adverse Effects
Blurred vision, dizziness, dry mouth, euphoria,
headache, nausea, pruritus, restlessness,
sedation, tachycardia, vomiting

**Special Nursing Considerations
and Patient Education**
• Protect medication from direct light.
• Reduce dose as quickly as possible.
• Observe for abdominal distention.
• Hold dose if electrolyte imbalance or dehydration
  occurs.
• Offer hard candy (regular or sugar-free) to relieve
  dry mouth.
• Administer medication only as directed,
  particularly liquid form.
• Be aware that
  – dependence is possible; when discontinued,
    decrease dose gradually.
• Teach patient
  – to be cautious when driving or involved in
    potentially hazardous tasks.

Dipyridamole

Brand Name
Persantine, Pyridamole

Actions
Antianginal, antiplatlet, coronary vasodilator.

Uses
Angina pectoris, prevention of coronary thrombosis, prevention of transient ischemic attacks, inhibition of platlet adhesion to prevent MI, thromboembolism

Contraindications
Hypersensitivity, hypotension. *Use with caution:* platlet defects

Interactions
Aspirin, NASAID, coumadin, heparin

Dose
Adult   PO: 75–100 mg qid

Forms
Tablets

Adverse Effects
Dizziness, abdominal stress, headache, rash, weakness, nausea, syncope, flushing

**Special Nursing Considerations
and Patient Education**
- Assess blood pressure lying and standing.
- Administer 1 hour prior to, or 2 hours after, meals.
- Evaluate chest pain.
- Provide safety measures for orthostatic
  hypotension.
- Provide small, frequent meals.
- Teach patient to
  - avoid driving.
  - change position slowly.
  - take as prescribed; do not double dose.
  - avoid alcohol and tobacco.

Doxepin HCl

Brand Name
Sinequan, Adapin

Actions
Tricyclic antidepressant; hinders reuptake of
norepinephrine. Onset evident in 2–3 weeks.

Uses
Anxiety, endogenous depression

Contraindications
Meds   Alcohol, MAO inhibitors
Other   Children under 12, narrow-angle glaucoma,
recent MI, urinary retention. *Use with
caution:* Cardiac dysfunction, diabetes,
epilepsy, glaucoma, hyperthyroidism,
prostatic hypertrophy

Interactions
Anticholinergics, clonidine, estrogen,
ethchlorvynol, guanethidine, hypnotics, levodopa,
narcotics, procainamide, quinidine, sedatives,
sympathomimetics, thyroid preparations,
tranquilizers

Dose
Adult   10–50 mg tid; additional effectiveness is
rarely obtained by exceeding 300 mg/day

Forms
Capsules, oral solution

Adverse Effects
Blurred vision, drowsiness, dry mouth,
extrapyramidal symptoms, decreased libido,
nausea, tinnitus, vomiting, weight gain

**Special Nursing Considerations
and Patient Education**
- Do not dilute concentrate with carbonated
  beverages; dilute in 120 ml of water.
- Use caution when administering to a patient with
  suicidal potential; ensure patient swallows dose.
- When discontinued, decrease dosage gradually.
- Offer hard candy (regular or sugar-free) to relieve
  dry mouth.
- Teach patient
    - to be cautious when driving or involved in
      potentially hazardous tasks.
    - that medication may cause a peculiar taste in
      mouth.
    - that it will take approximately 2–3 weeks before
      effect is felt.
    - to avoid CNS depressants, alcohol.

Doxycycline Hyclate

Brand Name
Vibramycin, Vibra-Tabs

Actions
Antiamebic, antibacterial, antibiotic, anti-infective, antirickettsial; hinders bacteria's formation of proteins. Onset evident in 1–2 hours.

Uses
Granuloma inguinale, lymphogranuloma, mycoplasma, ornithosis, psittacosis, rickettsial disease, spirochetal relapsing fever

Contraindications
Meds   Antacids, iron and mineral preparations
Other   Children. *Use with caution:* History of hepatic or renal dysfunction, lupus erythematosus

Interactions
Barbiturates, carbamazepine, methoxyflurane, oral anticoagulants, penicillin, phenytoin, sodium bicarbonate

Dose
Adult   PO: Initial dose: 200 mg in 2 divided doses; *maintenance* dose: 100 mg/day PO or IV infusion
Peds   PO: 100 lbs or less: initial dose, 4.4 mg/kg in 2 divided dose; *maintenance* dose: 2.2–4.4 mg/kg/day in 2 divided doses

142

Forms
Calcium salt syrup, hyclate capsules or injection,
monohydrate suspension

Adverse Effects
Diarrhea, dysphagia, jaundice, nausea, renal
impairment, superinfections, teeth discoloration
(children), vomiting

**Special Nursing Considerations
and Patient Education**
- Protect medication from light.
- Monitor urinary output.
- Teach patient
  - to continue medication for 24–48 hours after
    temperature returns to normal.
  - *not* to consume dairy products 1 hour before or
    after each dose, as they affect action of the
    medication.
  - to take dose 1 or 2 hours after eating.
  - that medication may cause photosensitivity.
  - to report to physician signs of superinfection:
    black, furry tongue, vaginal itching, rash.

Enalapril Maleate

Brand Names
Vasotec, Vasotec IV

Actions
Antihypertensive, angiotensin-converting enzyme inhibitor. Onset evident in 1 hour.

Uses
Hypertension

Contraindications
Hypersensitivity, severe hypotension, pregnancy, hyperkalemia

Interactions
Potassium (diet or drug), diuretics, aspirin, hypoglycemics, phenothiazines

Dose
Adult   PO: initial dose: 5 mg/day; may increase to 10–40 mg/day in divided doses; IV: 0.625 mg q6h

Forms
Tablets, injectables

Adverse Effects
Dizziness, hypotension, insomnia, urinary frequency, muscle cramps, nausea and vomiting, proteinuria

144

Special Nursing Considerations and Patient Education:

- Monitor vital signs every 4 hours.
- Instruct patient to move slowly because of possible orthostatic hypotension.
- Provide small, frequent meals if nausea occurs.
- Administer 1 hour prior to meals.
- Teach patient to
  - not take OTC medications without informing physician.
  - notify physician if edema, chest pain or irregular heartbeat occur.
  - not discontinue without physician's orders.

Erythromycin Base

Brand Name

E-Mycin, Eryc, AK-Mycin, Eryderm, Erymax, Ery-Tab, Ilotycin, Ilotycin Opthalmic, Robemycin, Robitabs, Staticin, T-Stat

Actions

Antibacterial. Onset evident: PO 1 hour; IV rapid.

Uses

Infections caused by: D. pneumoniae, M. Pneumoniae, C. diphtheriae, B. pertussis, L. monocytogenes, Legionella pneumophilia—URI, LRI, pelvic inflammatory disease, otitis media, chlamydia. Topic–acne vulgaris, minor skin abrasions.

Contraindications

Hypersensitivity. *Use with caution:* liver disease

Interactions

Sulfonamides, digoxin, oral anticoagulants, theophylline, cyclosporine, methylprednisolone, carbamazepine

Dose

Adult PO: 250 mg qid or 333 mg q8h; IV: 1–4 gm/day q6h

Peds PO: 30–50 mg/kg/day q6h; *maximum* dose: 100 mg/kg/day IV: 15–20 mg/kg/day in divided doses q6h

Forms
Tablets

Adverse Effects
Nausea and vomiting, diarrhea, abdominal pain,
cramping, rashes, superinfections, allergic
reactions, reversible hearing loss, uncontrollable
emotions, confusions, heartburn, anorexia,
tinnitus

**Special Nursing Considerations
and Patient Education**
- Administer around the clock on an empty
  stomach.
- May give with food if GI symptoms persist.
- Do not administer with fruit juice.
- Teach patient to
  - not crush or chew.
  - take with water.
  - report signs of superinfection.
  - take all of the medication.
  - notify physician if the symptoms persist.

Estradiol Transdermal System

Brand Name
Estraderm

Actions
Hormone

Uses
Moderate to severe vasomotor symptoms
associated with menopause, treatment of female
hypogonadism, female castration, primary ovarian
failure, atrophic conditions caused by deficient
endogenous estrogen production

Contraindications
Known or suspected carcinoma of the breast,
estrogen-dependent neoplasia, pregnancy,
undiagnosed abnormal genital bleeding,
thrombophlebitis or thromboembolic disorders,
history of thrombophlebitis or disorders
associated with previous estrogen use

Interactions
Increased sulfobromophthalein retention,
increased prothrombin time, increased thyroxine-
binding globulin, oral anticoagulants, tricyclic
antidepressants, insulin, barbiturates, phenytoin,
oral broad spectrum antibiotics

Dose
Adult   Apply 50 or 100mcg to skin twice weekly. (If
on oral estrogen, begin 1 week after withdrawal from oral therapy). 3 weeks on, 1
week off.

Forms
Patch

Adverse Effects
Irritation at application site, breakthrough
bleeding, spotting, change in menstrual flow,
change in cervical secretion, breast tenderness,
breast enlargement, nausea, vomiting, abdominal
cramps, bloating, intolerance to contact lenses,
headache, dizziness, weight change, edema,
libido change

**Special Nursing Considerations
and Patient Education**
• Do not apply to breasts, waistline.
• Rotate site of applications, with 1 week between
applications.
• Inform patient that bathing and swimming will not
affect system.
• Follow 3 weeks on, 1 week off regimen.
• Apply to clean, dry area; apply and press for 10
seconds.
• Teach patient to
  – apply immediately upon removal from package.
  – notify physician of suspected pregnancy.

Estrogens, Conjugated

Brand Name
Premarin

Actions
Similar to endogenous estrogen; synthesis of selected proteins and RNA

Uses
Breast or prostatic cancer palliation, dysfunctional uterine hemorrhage, hypogonadism (female), kraurosis or pruritus vulvae, postpartum breast engorgement, senile vaginitis, vasomotor symptoms of menopause, possible prevention of post menopausal osteoporosis

Contraindications
Estrogen-dependent neoplasia, pregnancy, thromboembolic disorders, undiagnosed vaginal bleeding. *Use with caution:* Asthma, cardiac or renal dysfunction, children, epilepsy, jaundice, metabolic bone disease, migraine headache

Interactions
Tricyclic antidepressants

Dose
Adult   PO: 0.3–1.25 mg/day; IV/IM: 25 mg q6–12 hrs; intravaginal: cream, 2–4 gm/day
Peds   Adolescent: Individualized: 5–10 mg

150

Forms
Cream, injection, tablets

Adverse Effects
Abdominal cramps, chloasma, chorea, headache,
hirsutism, menstrual abnormalities, nausea,
vaginal hemorrhage, vomiting

**Special Nursing Considerations
and Patient Education**
- Store in refrigerator.
- Be aware that
  - medication may increase risk of endometrial
    carcinoma, gallbladder disease, MI, pulmonary
    embolism, thrombophlebitis.
- Teach patient to
  - notify physician of suspected pregnancy.
  - decrease smoking.
  - notify physician if chest or leg pain or vaginal
    bleeding occur.

Ethchlorvynol

Brand Name
Placidyl

Actions
Anticonvulsant, CNS depressant, hypnotic,
muscle relaxant. Onset evident in 30 minutes.

Uses
Anxiety, insomnia, tension, to achieve sedation

Contraindications
Meds   Alcohol, CNS depressants
Other   Children, history of porphyria. *Use with
caution:* Hepatic or renal dysfunction,
uncontrolled pain

Interactions
Antihistamines, hypnotics, MAO inhibitors,
narcotics, oral anticoagulants, sedatives, tricyclic
antidepressants, tranquilizers

Dose
Adult   100 mg–1 gm hs

Forms
Capsules

Adverse Effects
Blurred vision, dizziness, facial numbness, headache, hives, hypotension, nausea, urticaria, vomiting

Special Nursing Considerations Patient Education
- Store medication in light-resistant container.
- If used as a hypnotic, administer 15–30 minutes prior to bedtime.
- Discontinue for hemorrhage, rash.
- Use caution when administering to a patient with suicidal potential; ensure patient swallows dose.
- Be aware that
  - medication may be habit-forming; when discontinued, decrease dosage gradually.
  - tolerance can develop.
- Teach patient
  - that medication may cause aftertaste, pale stools, dark urine.
  - to be cautious when driving or involved in potentially hazardous tasks.

Famotidine

Brand Name
Pepcid

Actions
H_2 Histimine antagonist. Onset evident in 1 hour.

Uses
Short-term treatment of active duodenal ulcer, maintenance therapy for duodenal ulcer, Zollinger-Ellison syndrome, multiple endocrine adenomas

Contraindications
Hypersensitivity

Interactions
None

Dose
Adult   PO: active duodenal ulcer: 40 mg qhs; maintenance therapy for duodenal ulcer: 20 mg qhs IV: 20 mg q12h; hypersecretory conditions: PO: 20 mg q6h; IV: 20 mg q12h Administer IV: 2ml pepcid/100ml IV solution; rate: 15–30 minutes.

Forms
Tablets, injection

Adverse Effects
Headache, dizziness, constipation, diarrhea, abdominal pain, muscle cramps, rash, sexual impotence

Special Nursing Considerations and Patient Education
- Administer at hs.
- Arrange for blood tests for follow-up evaluation.
- Teach patient to
    - be aware that possible decreased libido is reversible after the medication is discontinued.
    - report signs of blood dyscrasias: brusing, bleeding, fatigue.
    - shake oral suspension prior to use.
    - discard oral suspension after 30 days.

Flunisolide

Brand Name
Aerobid, Nasalide

Actions
Corticosteroid. Onset evident within 3 weeks.

Uses
Topical treatment of seasonal or perennial rhinitis, nasal polyps

Contraindications
Hypersensitivity, active or quiescent tuberculosis infections of respiratory tract, ocular herpes simplex, untreated systemic viral, fungal or bacterial infections. *Use with caution*: nasal ulcers, recurrent epistaxis, nasal surgery

Interactions
Systemic corticosteroids

Dose
Adult   2 sprays/nostril bid-tid, not to exceed 8 sprays/nostril/day
Ped   1 spray/nostril tid or 2 sprays/bid; not to exceed 4 sprays/nostril/day

Forms
Nasal spray bottle

Adverse Effects

Transient nasal burning/stinging, nasal congestion, sneezing, epistaxis, watery eyes, sore throat, headaches, altered sense of smell and taste, Cushing's syndrome

Special Nursing Considerations and Patient Education

- Administer lowest effective dose.
- Teach patient to
  - use spray at regular intervals.
  - use as directed only.
  - be aware that therapeutic effects may take up to 1–2 weeks.
  - use spray bottle properly.

Fluoxetine

Brand Name
Prozac

Actions
Antidepressant. Onset evident: within 4 weeks;
peaks in 6–8 hours.

Uses
Major depressive disorders

Contraindications
None known. *Use with caution*: metabolic or
hemodynamic conditions

Interactions
MAO inhibitors, diazepam, L-trytophan

Dose
Adult   PO: initial dose: 20 mg qam; may increase
to 20 mg bid; *maximum* dose: 80 mg/day

Forms
Pulvules

Adverse Effects
Headache, nervousness, insomnia, drowsiness,
anxiety, tremors, dizziness, fatigue, decreased
libido, decreased concentration, nausea, diarrhea,
dry mouth, anorexia, dyspepsia, constipation,
excessive sweating, asthenia, viral infection, URI,

nasal congestion, sinusitis, back pain, vision
disturbances, sedation, chills, change in appetite,
hot flashes, dysmenorrhea, urinary frequency,
urinary tract infection, abnormal dreams, weight
loss, agitation, bronchitis, rhinitis

Special Nursing Considerations
and Patient Education
- Be aware that therapeutic effect takes 2–3 weeks.
- Be certain that patient swallows the medication.
- Evaluate for history of drug abuse.
- Assess mental status, including suicidal
  tendencies, during treatment.
- Assess weight every week.
- Administer with food or milk to decrease GI
  disturbances.
- Administer at hs if sedative effect occurs.
- Provide hard candy and water to relieve dry
  mouth.
- Provide safety measures as needed.
- Teach patient to
  - have periodic evaluations by physician to
    determine the effectiveness of the medication.
  - avoid driving, operating machinery.
  - avoid alcohol and OTC medications.
  - notify physician of suspected pregnancy.
  - not discontinue the medication without
    physician's approval.

Flurazepam HCl

Brand Name
Dalmane

Actions
Hypnotic. Onset evident in 30–60 minutes.

Uses
Insomnia (short-term)

Contraindications
Meds Alcohol
Other Children under 15, depression, hepatic or
renal dysfunction. *Use with caution:* Allergy
to chemically related medications, epilepsy,
pulmonary disease

Interactions
Anticonvulsants, antidepressants, CNS
depressants, hypnotics, MAO inhibitors, narcotics,
sedatives, tranquilizers, tricyclic antidepressants

Dose
Adult 15–30 mg hs
Peds Over 15 years: Same as adult

Forms
Capsules

160

Adverse Effects
Ataxia, diarrhea, dizziness, headache, lightheadedness, nausea, sedation, vomiting

**Special Nursing Considerations
and Patient Education**
- Protect medication from heat and direct light.
- Provide safety measures.
- Be aware that
  - effects may be cumulative.
  - dependence is possible; when discontinued,
    decrease dosage gradually.
- Teach patient
  - to decrease use of caffeine and cigarettes/
    cigars because of their stimulating effect.
  - to be cautious when driving or involved in
    potentially hazardous tasks.
  - to avoid CNS depressants, alcohol.

Flurbiprofen

Brand Name
Ansaid

Actions
Nonsteroidal anti-inflammatory, analgesic, antipyretic. Onset evident within 1 month.

Uses
Rheumatoid arthritis, osteoarthritis

Contraindications
Hypersensitivity. *Use with caution*: bleeding disorders, cardiac dissorders, GI disorders, severe renal or hepatic disease.

Interactions
Anticoagulants, phenytoin, sulfonamides, sulfonylureas, aspirin, beta-blockers

Dose
Adult   PO: 200–300 mg in divided doses bid-qid

Forms
Tablets

Adverse Effects
Nausea, vomiting, diarrhea, dizziness, tremors, confusion, tachycardia, rash, dry mouth, blurred vision, shortness of breath, tinnitus

**Special Nursing Considerations
and Patient Education**

- Assess blood, liver and renal studies prior to and during treatment.
- Administer on empty stomach if possible.
- Teach patient to
  - notify physician if blurred vision or tinnitus occur.
  - be aware that therapeutic effects may take up to 1 month.
  - avoid alcohol and aspirin.
  - avoid OTC medications.
  - take with food or milk to decrease GI discomfort.

Furosemide

Brand Name
Lasix

Actions
Diuretic; hinders chloride and sodium reabsorption. Onset evident: PO 20–60 minutes; IV 5 minutes, IM 10–30 minutes.

Uses
Ascites, cirrhosis, congestive heart failure, nephrosis, pulmonary edema, renal dysfunction

Contraindications
Anuria, electrolyte depletion, jaundice (children, infants), oliguria, renal dysfunction. *Use with caution:* Allergy to sulfonamides, diabetes, gout, hearing impairment, hepatic dysfunction, hyperuricemia, lupus erythematosus, pancreatitis

Interactions
Alcohol, amikacin, capreomycin, chloroquine, ethacrynic acid, kanamycin, lithium, neomycin, ototoxic drugs, oxyphenbutazone, phenyl-butazone, streptomycin, vancomycin, viomycin

Dose
Adult PO: 20–80 mg as single dose in morning (dosage may be carefully titrated up to 600 mg/day); IM, IV: 20–40 mg as single dose in morning

Peds   PO: 2 mg/kg/day; IM, IV: 1 mg/kg/day;
         maximum dose: 6 mg /kg/day

Forms
Injection, liquid, tablets

Adverse Effects
Blurred vision, diarrhea, hyperuricemia,
hypokalemia, hyponatremia, muscle cramps,
nausea, paresthesia, orthostatic hypotension,
transient deafness, vomiting

**Special Nursing Considerations
and Patient Education**
- Protect medication from direct light.
- Administer IV Dose slowly over 1–2 minutes.
- Inject IM dose slowly into deep muscles.
- Observe for hypersensitivity to sulfonamides
  (patients may experience cross-allergenicity).
- Monitor blood pressure; blood levels of carbon
  dioxide, electrolytes, serum BUN; I&0; vital signs;
  weight.
- Discontinue for hearing impairment, hypokalemia,
  hyponatremia.
- Be aware that
  – patient may need potassium supplements or
    changes in salt intake.
- Teach patient
  – that medication may cause sweet taste in
    mouth.

- to change position slowly to decrease postural hypotension.
- to be cautious during hot weather or strenuous exercise to decrease possibility of orthostatic hypotension.
- to follow high-potassium diet.

Notes

Gemfibrozil

Brand Name
Lopid

Actions
Inhibits peripheral lipolysis. Lipid-regulating agent which decreases serum triglyceride resulting in decreased total-serum cholesterol. Onset evident in 1–2 hours.

Uses
Hyperlipidemia—Type IV & V

Contraindications
Severe hepatic disease, allergy, renal dysfunction, primary biliary
cirrhosis, gall bladder disease

Interactions
Anticoagulants

Dose
Adult PO: 1200 mg in divided doses bid ½ hour before meals

Forms
Capsules, tablets

Adverse Effects

Abdominal pain, epigastric pain, nausea, vomiting,
diarrhea, flatulence, dry mouth, constipation, rash,
dermatitis, headache, dizziness, blurred vision,
painful extremities, cholelithiasis, swollen joints,
impairment of fertility, vertigo, anorexia, back pain

Special Nursing Considerations and Patient Education

- Administer with meals to decrease GI discomfort.
- Monitor nutritional status.
- Refer to dietician.
- Assess renal and hepatic fucntion if therapy is long-term.
- Teach patient to
  - follow low-cholesterol diet, exercise program.
  - use caution while driving.
  - take medication as directed.
  - use birth control while on medication.

Glipizide

Brand Name
Glucotrol

Actions
Antidiabetic. Onset evident in 15–30 minutes.

Uses
Non-insulin dependent diabetes mellitus

Contraindications
Hypersensitivity, insulin-dependent diabetes mellitus, severe kidney/liver/thyroid/endocrine dysfunction, severe infections, severe trauma, major surgery

Interactions
Alcohol, digitoxin, insulin, MAO inhibitors, cimetidine, calcium channel blockers, corticosteroids, oral contraceptives, thiazide diuretics, estrogen, phenothiazines, phenytoin, rifampin, probenecid, thyroid products, nonsteroidal anti-inflammatory agents

Dose
Adult: PO: 2.5–40 mg/day; administer doses greater than 20 mg in divided doses bid; *maximum* dose: 40 mg/day.

Forms
Tablets

Adverse Effects
Headache, weakness, dizziness, drowsiness,
cholestatic jaundice, nausea, vomiting,
hypoglycemia, pruritis, urticaria, leukopenia,
photosensitivity, diarrhea

**Special Nursing Considerations
and Patient Education**
- Observe for signs and symptoms of
  hypoglycemia.
- May administer with meals or 30 minutes before.
- May crush tablets.
- Inform the patient that this medication does not
  cure diabetes mellitus.
- Refer to dietician.
- Monitor serum glucose.
- Provide good skin care.
- Teach patient to
  - recognize signs and symptoms of hypoglycemia
    and treatment.
  - take medication at the same time every day.
  - not take alcohol or OTC medications.
  - test urine or serum glucose as directed.
  - follow diabetic regimen (diet, exercise, hygiene).
  - not discontinue medication abruptly.

Glyberride

Brand Name
DiaBeta, Micronase

Actions
Oral hypoglycemic. Onset evident in 30–45 minutes.

Uses
Non-insulin dependent diabetes mellitus

Contraindications
Hypersensitivity, diabetic ketoacidosis with or without coma, severe renal or hepatic disease, brittle diabetes, juvenile diabetes, endocrine dysfunction. *Use with caution*: history of cardiac disease

Interactions
Alcohol, salicylates, sulfonamides, chloramphenicol, probenecid, coumaius, MAO inhibitors, thiazides, diuretics, phenotiazines, estrogens, oral contraceptives, phenytoin, nicotinic acid, corticosteroids, dicumarol, beta-adrenergic blocking agents, calcium channel blockers

Dose
Adult　PO: initial dose: 2.5–5 mg qd; *maintenance* dose: 1.25–20 mg qd

Forms
Tablets

Adverse Effects
Hypoglycemia, nausea, epigastric fullness,
heartburn, pruritus, erythema, urticaria,
maculopapular erruptions, photosensitivity,
leukopenia, headache, weakness, cholestatic
jaundice, dizziness

**Special Nursing Considerations
and Patient Education**
- Administer every AM with breakfast.
- May crush tablets.
- Observe for signs and symptoms of
  hypoglycemia.
- If GI upset occurs, may divide dose.
- Arrange for insulin prn (infections, trauma,
  surgery).
- Monitor diet; refer to dietician.
- Help patient understand that the medication does
  not cure diabetes.
- Provide good skin care.
- Teach patient to
  - follow diabetic regimen (diet, exercise, hygiene).
  - know signs and symptoms of hypoglycemia and
    treatment.
  - monitor serum glucose or urine glucose.
  - not take alcohol or OTC medications with
    alcohol.
  - use sunscreen.
  - not discontinue medication abruptly.

173

Glyburide

Brand Name
Micronase, DiaBeta

Actions
Antidiabetic. Onset evident in 45–60 minutes.

Uses
Non-insulin dependent diabetes mellitus, onset of diabetes mellitus in stable adult

Contraindications
Hypersensitivity. Diabetes mellitus–insulin-dependent, juvenile onset, brittle, ketosis-prone, type I

Interactions
Insulin, MAO inhibitors, anti-inflammatory agents, salicylates, sulfonamides, alcohol, glucocorticoids, thiazide diuretics, oral anticoagulants, beta-adrenergic blocking agents, thyroid preparations, phenothiazines, phenytoin, rifampin

Dose
Adult   PO: initial dose: 2.5–5.0 mg; PO: 1.25–20 mg single dose >10 mg, divide bid. Maintenance dose: 1.25–20.0 mg/day; *maximum* dose: 20 mg/day; administer once a day or divide bid

Forms
Tablets

Adverse Effects
Hypoglycemia, nausea, heartburn, epigastric fullness, pruritus, erythema, uticaria, leukopenia, headache, weakness, fever, jaundice, dizziness, drowsiness, photosensitivity

**Special Nursing Considerations
and Patient Education**
- Administer 30 minutes before meals (breakfast).
- Observer for signs and symptoms of jaundice— yellow sceleras, dark urine.
- Test urine glucose levels tid.
- Observe for signs and symptoms of hypo- and hyperglycemia.
- Teach patient to
  - be aware of signs and symptoms of hypo- and hyperglycemia.
  - take an daily basis; not discontinue the medication abruptly.
  - take medication before breakfast.
  - follow ADA diet as prescribed.
  - not take medication if unable to eat.
  - avoid alcohol, OTC medications.
  - utilize sunscreen.

Guaifenesin/Theophylline

Brand Name
Quibron

Actions
Bronchodilator, expectorant, sympathomimetic.
Onset evident in 1 hour.

Uses
Asthmatic bronchospasm, chronic bronchitis,
emphysema

Contraindications
Hypersensitivity. *Use with caution:* Acute cardiac
disease, cor pulmonale, glaucoma, gout, hepatic
or renal disease, hypertension, hyperthyroidism,
hypoxemia, myocardial damage, neonates,
porphyria, prostatic hypertrophy

Interactions
Allopurinol, anticoagulants, chlordiazepoxide,
cimetidine, clindamycin, digitalis, erythromycin,
furosemide, lincomycin, lithium, phenobarbital,
phenytoin, propranolol, sympathomimetics

Dose
Adult 150 mg q6–8h or 15–30 cc q6h
Peds Under 9 yr: 4–6 mg of theophylline/kg q6–
8h; 9–12 yr: 4–5 mg of theophylline/kg q6–
8h

Forms
   Capsules, liquid

Adverse Effects
   CNS stimulation, dizziness, gastric upset,
   headache, insomnia, nausea, tachycardia,
   vomiting

**Special Nursing Considerations
and Patient Education**
- Monitor I&O, vital signs.
- Administer after meals and with a glass of water
  to decrease GI irritation.
- Teach patient to
   - be cautious when driving or involved in
     potentially hazardous tasks.
   - not take OTC medications without conferring
     with physician.
   - decrease intake of caffeine.

Guanfacine Hydrochloride

Brand Name
Tenex

Actions
Antihypertensive

Uses
Moderate to severe hypertension

Contraindications
Hypersensitivity. *Use with caution*: CNS
depressants

Interactions
CNS depressants

Dose
Adult PO: 1 mg hs; may increase after 3–4
weeks to 2–3 mg hs

Forms
Tablets

Adverse Effects
Dry mouth, somnolence, dizziness, constipation,
fatigue, headache, insomnia, impotence

Special Nursing Considerations
and Patient Education

- Monitor blood pressure prior to and during treatment.
- Assess edema,I&O, weight.
- Assess for CHF signs.
- Teach patient to
  - avoid alcohol, OTC medications.
  - not discontinue medication abruptly.

Haloperidol

Brand Name
Haldol

Actions
Antipsychotic; inhibits brainstem activity. Onset evident: PO 3 weeks; IM 30–45 minutes.

Uses
Acute or chronic psychotic disorders, behavioral problems, Gilles de la Tourette's syndrome

Contraindicitions
Meds Alcohol, CNS depressants, lithium
Other Children under 3 years, comatose patients, depression, parkinsonism. *Use with caution:* Cardiovascular, hepatic or respiratory dysfunction; diabetes; epilepsy; glaucoma

Interactions
Anticonvulsants, antihistamines, barbiturates, guanethidine, hypnotics, narcotics, oral anticoagulants, sedatives, tranquilizers, tricyclic antidepressants

Dose
Adult PO: 0.5–5 mg bid–tid; IM: 2–5 mg q1–8h; individualized doses up to 100 mg may be necessary.
Peds Over 3 yr: 0.05–0.15 mg/kg/day PO

Forms
Concentrate, injection, tablets

Adverse Effects
Blurred vision, constipation, drowsiness, dry
mouth, extrapyramidal symptoms, headache,
insomnia, nausea, orthostatic hypotension,
tachycardia, vomiting

**Special Nursing Considerations
and Patient Education**
- Protect medication from direct light.
- Monitor for fine vermicular tongue movements
  (may indicate early tardive dyskinesia).
- Dilute concentrate in fluids other than coffee or
  tea; do not dilute if possible.
- Give injections in upper, outer quadrant of
  buttocks.
- Have patient lie down for 1 hour after parenteral
  administration.
- Monitor blood pressure.
- Discontinue for jaundice, tremors, impairment or
  weakness of vision.
- Be aware that
  – medication is eliminated slowly.
  – medication decreases seizure threshold.
- Teach patient
  – to be cautious when driving or involved in
    potentially hazardous tasks.
  – to use caution when in the sun because of the
    possibility of photosensitivity.
  – to change position slowly.

Heparin Sodium Injection

Brand Name
Hep-Lock, Lipo-Hepin

Actions
Anticoagulant; hinders prothrombin from forming thrombin. Onset evident: sc 20–60 minutes; IV immediate.

Uses
Arterial occlusion; atrial fibrillation with embolism; cardiac/vascular surgery; hyperlipemia; pulmonary embolism; thrombophlebitis; adjunct treatment of coronary occlusion with acute MI

Contraindications
Meds   Anesthetics (lumber block , regional)
Other   Acute hemorrhage; blood dycrasias; chronic ulcerative colitis; following brain, eye, or spinal cord surgery; hepatic or renal dysfunction; hypertension; peptic ulcer; shock; subacute bacterial endocarditis; suspected intracranial hemorrhage; threatened abortion; tube drainage of small intestine and stomach; visceral carcinoma. *Use with caution:* Alcoholism, allergies, arteriosclerosis, asthma, indwelling catheter, jaundice, menstruation, open wounds, ACTH, antihistamines, aspirin, corticosteroids, dextran, diazepam, digitalis, purpura, skin denudation, thrombocytopenia, thrombophlebitis, ulcerative lesions

Interactions
dipyridamole, hydroxychloroquine, ibuprofen,
    indomethacin, insulin, tetracycline

Dose
Adult   IV infusion: 10,000–40,000 U/day; SC–deep:
          initially, 10,000–20,000 U, then 8,000–
          10,000 U q8h
Peds   IV infusion: 50 U/kg; followed by 100 U/kg or
          3,333 U/M² 6×/day

Forms
    Injection, pre-filled syringes

Adverse Effects
    Alopecia, chills, ecchymosis, epistaxis, fever,
    hemarthrosis, hematuria, hemorrhage

**Special Nursing Considerations
and Patient Education**
• Use trial dose to test for allergic response.
• Verify clotting time, PTT, or APTT prior to
  administration (dosage is adjusted according to
  these lab values).
• Avoid IM route since there is a tendency for
  patient to form hematomas.
• Administer SC via Z-track technique. Do not rub
  skin before or after SC injection as this may
  damage tissue. Do not pinch skin or withdraw
  plunger before administration.
• Monitor clotting time, vital signs; check injection
  site, stools, and urine for bleeding.

- Be aware that
  - patient is in increased danger of hemorrhage.
- Teach patient to
  - not smoke.
  - carry some type of Medic Alert bracelet or card containing dosage and resource telephone numbers.
  - notify physician of any signs of hemorrhage.

Notes

Hydrochlorothiazide

Brand Name
Esidrix, HydroDIURIL, Oretic

Actions
Antihypertensive, diuretic; hinders sodium
reabsorption. Onset evident in 2 hours.

Uses
Edema, hypertension

Contraindications
Meds Lithium
Other Hypersensitivity to sulfonamide-derived
medications, renal decompensation. *Use
with caution:* Allergy to sulfonamides,
diabetes, gout, hepatic or renal dysfunction,
hypercalcemia, hyperuricemia, lupus
erythematosus, pancreatitis, sympathectomy

Interactions
ACTH, antigout drugs, antihypertensives,
corticosteroids, digitalis, insulin, lithium, oral
antidiabetics

Dose
Adult Edema: 25–200 mg qd; hypertension: 75
mg/day, to be adjusted
Peds Under 6 month: 3.3 mg/kg/day in 2 doses;
over 6 months: 2.2 mg/kg/day

Forms
Tablets

Adverse Effects
Anorexia, constipation, diarrhea, dizziness, headache, hypokalemia, hypotension, nausea, orthostatic hypotension, paresthesia, vomiting

Special Nursing Considerations And Patient Education

- Monitor blood pressure, electrolytes (particularly serum potassium level), weight, I&O
- Discontinue for electrolyte imbalances.
- Administer in AM.
- Teach patient
  - that medication may cause photosensitivity.
  - to ingest potassium-rich foods (see Appendix F).
  - to be cautious when driving or involved in potentially hazardous tasks.
  - to use caution during hot weather or strenuous exercise because of the possibility of orthostatic hypotension.
  - to follow hypertension regime: stress management, weight reduction, exercise.

Hydroflumethiazide/Reserpine

Brand Name
Salutensin

Actions
Antihypertensive, diuretic; hinders reabsorption of
sodium and chloride in tubules

Uses
Hypertension

Contraindications
Active peptic ulcer, anuria, children, depression,
ECT, oliguria, ulcerative colitis. *Use with caution:*
Asthma, diabetes, digitalized patients, gallstones,
GI disorders, gout, hyperuricemia, lupus
erythematosus, renal insufficiency

Interactions
ACTH, anticonvulsants, antihistamines, digitalis,
hypnotics, insulin, MAO inhibitors, narcotics, oral
anticoagulants, phenothiazines, propranolol,
quinidine, sedatives, steroids, tranquilizers

Dose
Adult   Individualized; *average* dose: 1–2 tablets
            qd–bid

Forms
Demi-tablets, tablets

Adverse Effects
Anorexia, constipation, depression, diarrhea, dizziness, drowsiness, dry mouth, dyspnea, electrolyte and fluid imbalance, hypokalemia, hypotension, lethargy, nasal congestion, nausea, restlessness, syncope, tachycardia, thirst, vertigo, vomiting

Special Nursing Considerations and Patient Education
- Protect medication from direct light.
- Monitor blood pressure, I&O, pulse, weight.
- Offer hard candy (regular or sugar-free) to relieve dry mouth.
- Administer with meals or milk to decrease GI upset.
- Consult with physician regarding diet.
- Be aware that
  - generally, this drug is not used for initial therapy.
- Teach patient
  - that medication may cause photosensitivity.
  - to be cautious when driving or involved in potentially hazardous tasks.
  - to change position slowly to decrease hypotension.
  - to not take nonprescription medications without conferring with physician.

Hydroxyzine HCl, Hydroxyzine Pamoate

Brand Name
Atarax, Vistaril

Actions
Anticholinergic, antiemetic, antihistamine, sedative, tranquilizer; depresses brainstem (reticular formation) and hypothalamus. Onset evident in 15–30 minutes.

Uses
Allergic dermatoses, anxiety, nausea, psychomotor agitation, tension, urticaria

Contraindications
Alcohol, CNS depressants. *Use with caution:* Epilepsy

Interactions
Analgesics, anticholinesterase drugs, anticoagulants, antihistamines, barbiturates, hypnotics, narcotics, phenothiazines, sedatives

Dose
Adult PO: 25–100 mg tid–qid
Peds Under 6 yr: 50 mg/day PO in divided doses
Over 6 yr: 50–100 mg/day PO in divided doses

Forms
Hydroxyzine hydrochloride capsules, Injections,
syrup, and tablets; hydroxyzine pamoate
capsules, injection, and suspension

Adverse Effects
Drowsiness, dry mouth, headache, tremors

**Special Nursing Considerations
and Patient Education**
- Protect medication from light.
- Shake suspension well prior to administering.
- Administer IM Injections slowly into deep muscles
  (buttocks for adults, midlateral thigh for children)
  to prevent nerve injury; rotate sites.
- Be aware that
  - tolerance can develop.
- Teach patient to
  - be cautious when driving or involved in
    potentially hazardous tasks.
  - decrease caffeine intake because of its
    stimulant effect.

Ibuprofen

Brand Name
Motrin, Advil

Actions
Analgesic, anti-inflammatory, antipyretic. Onset
evident in 1 hour.

Uses
Menstrual pain, osteoarthritis, rheumatoid arthritis

Contraindications
Allergy to aspirin, anglodermatitis, aspirin-induced
bronchospasm, children under 14, nasal polyps.
Use with caution: Cardiovascular
decompensation, coagulation disorders,
congestive heart failure, peptic ulcer, renal
dysfunction, upper GI tract disorders.

Interactions
Alcohol, anticoagulants, aspirin, phenobarbital,
phenytoin, sulfonamides, sulfonylureas

Dose
Adult 300–400 mg tid–qid; *maximum* dose: 2,400
mg/day

Forms
Tablets

Adverse Effects
Blurred vision, constipation, cramps, diarrhea, dizziness, dyspepsia, headache, pruritus, tinnitus

Special Nursing Considerations and Patient Education
- Administer medication with food to decrease GI distress.
- Monitor level of pain prior to and during administration.
- Teach patient
  - to be cautious when driving or involved in potentially hazardous tasks.
  - notify physician for blurred vision, edema, skin rash, tarry stools, weight gain.
  - to remain upright for 15–30 minutes.

Imipramine HCl

Brand Name
Tofranil

Actions
Antidepressant, antipsychotic; hinders re-uptake
of norepinephrine

Uses
Endogenous or manic depression, involutional
psychoses

Contraindications
Meds   Alcohol, MAO inhibitors
Other   Narrow-angle glaucoma, recent MI. *Use with
caution:* Alcoholism, asthma, cardiovascular
or hepatic dysfunction, diabetes, epilepsy,
glaucoma, hyperthyroidism, intraocular
pressure increase, prostatic hypertrophy,
urinary retention

Interactions
Amphetamines, anticholinergics, anticonvulsants.
antihistamines, antihypertensives, barbiturates,
clonidine, CNS depressants, estrogens,
ethchlorvynol, guanethidine, hypnotics, levodopa,
narcotics, quinidine, sedatives, sympathomimetics, thyroid preparations, tranquilizers

Dose
Adult   PO: 50 mg bid; Increase to *maximum* of 200
mg/day
Peds   PO: 25 mg/day 1 hr before hs

194

Forms
Injection, tablets

Adverse Effects
Anorexia, blurred vision, bone-marrow
depression, disorientation, dizziness, drowsiness,
dry mouth, dysrhythmias, hallucinations,
headache, nausea, paresthesia, seizures,
tachycardia, urinary retention, vomiting

**Special Nursing Considerations
and Patient Education**
- Protect medication from light.
- Monitor I&O, vital signs, weight.
- Use caution when administering to a patient with
  suicidal potential; ensure patient swallows dose.
- Offer hard candy (regular or sugar-free) to relieve
  dry mouth.
- Be aware that
  - tolerance can develop; when discontinued,
    decrease dosage gradually.
- Teach patient
  - to change position slowly to decrease
    hypotension.
  - to be cautious when driving or involved in
    potentially hazardous tasks.
  - that medication may cause a peculiar taste in
    mouth or photosensitivity.
  - to not take any nonprescription drugs without
    notifying physician.

Indapamide

Brand Name
Lozol

Actions
Antihypertsensive, diuretic. Onset evident in 1–2 hours.

Uses
Hypertension, edema due to CHF

Contraindications
Hypersensitivity, anuria. *Use with caution:* renal or hepatic impairment, hyperkalemia, dehydration, ascites, systemic lupus erythematosus

Interactions
Other antihypertensives, lithium, diazoxide, MAO inhibitors, alcohol, narcotics, barbiturates, muscle relaxants, steroids

Dose
Adult   PO: 2.5mg qam; may increase to 5.0 mg qd

Forms
Tablets

Adverse Effects
Headache, dizziness, fatigue, loss of energy,
muscle cramps, nervousness, extremity
numbness, anxiety, vertigo, depression, insomnia,
blurred vision, nausea, vomiting, constipation,
abdominal cramps, orthostatic hypotension,
urinary frequency, nocturia, rash, rhinorrhea

**Special Nursing Considerations
and Patient Education**
- Monitor blood pressure both lying and standing.
- Monitor weight, I&O daily.
- Administer qam.
- Assess for edema.
- Schedule follow-up appointments.
- Teach patient to
  - change position slowly.
  - take with food or milk.
  - follow prescribed diet; exercise and begin
    stress-management program.
  - not take OTC medications.

Indomethacin

Brand Name
Indocin

Actions
Analgesic, anti-inflammatory, antipyretic; blocks prostaglandin biosynthesis. Onset evident in 4–24 hours.

Uses
Degenerative joint disease of the hip, gout, gouty or rheumatoid arthritis, rheumatoid spondylitis

Contraindications
Active gastritis, children, enteritis, ileitis, nasal polyps associated with aspirin hypersensitivity, peptic ulcer, ulcerative colitis. *Use with caution;* Epilepsy, GI disorders, hemophilia, mental illness, parkinsonism, renal disease

Interactions
Aspirin, corticosteroids, furosemide, oral anticoagulants, phenylbutazone, probenicid, salicylates, sulfonamides, thyroid preparations

Dose
Adult   25 mg bid-tid

Forms
Capsules

Adverse Effects
Blurred vision, diarrhea, dizziness, drowsiness, headache, nausea, vomiting

Special Nursing Considerations and Patient Education
- Protect medication from direct light.
- Teach patient
  - to be cautious when driving or involved in potentially hazardous tasks.
  - to take with antacids, food, or after meals to decrease stomach irritation.
  - that this is a toxic medication and to take exactly as directed.
  - to notify physician for blurred vision or tarry stools.
  - to avoid salicylates, alcohol.

Insulin

Brand Name
Iletin (Regular), Iletin II (Regular), Insulin (Regular)

Actions
Antidiabetic, antihyperglycemic; necessary for amino acid and monosaccharide molecule transport. Onset evident in ½-1 hour.

Uses
Diabetes, diabetic coma

Contraindications
None. *Use with caution:* Fever, hepatic or renal dysfunction, hyper- or hypothyroidism, infections, nausea, vomiting

Interactions
Alcohol, anabolic steroids, corticosteroids, epinephrine, guanethidine, MAO Inhibitors, oral contraceptives, phenylbutazone, propranolol, sulfinpyrazone, tetracycline, thiazide diuretics, thyroid replacement

Dose
Adult Individualized; *average* dose: 50–150 U/day
Peds Individualized; *average* dose: 1–4 U/kg/day

Forms
Injection

Adverse Effects
Anxiety, diaphoresis, hypersensitivity or resistance to insulin, hypoglycemia, lassitude, nausea, tremulousness, visual disturbances

**Special Nursing Considerations
and Patient Education**
- Protect medication from heat and light.
- Check expiration date on label.
- Follow administration directions precisely.
- Verify that syringe gradations are aprropriate to strength of insulin preparation.
- Administer injections SC into loose connective tissue.
- Refrigerate stock supply
- Recognize the difference between this type and other types of insulin.
- Be aware that
  - insulin vial currently in use is stable at room temperature up to 1 month.
  - medication should be clear as water.
  - 1 unit of insulin will promote metabolism of approximately 1.5 gm of dextrose.
- Mix with other insulins as follows:
  - Lente Insulin (1:1): mix immediately prior to administration
  - NPH Insulin (any ratio): mix immediately prior to administration
  - Protamine Zinc (any ratio): prepare mixture immediately prior to injection.

- Teach patient
  - to maintain prescribed fluid intake and diet.
  - to carry sugar at all times.
  - to self-test urine.
  - to self-administer medication; ask for return demonstration.
  - that medication must be taken as directed and carried on person when traveling.
  - to use caution during strenuous exercise; dosage adjustment may be required.
  - to maintain good personal hygiene to prevent infections
  - to notify physician of illness.
  - to not take any new medications without contacting physician.
  - to carry some type of Medic Alert card or bracelet.

Notes

_____

_____

_____

_____

_____

_____

_____

_____

_____

_____

_____

_____

_____

_____

_____

_____

_____

Ipratropium Bromide

Brand Name
Atrovent

Actions
Anticholinergic

Uses
Bronchodilator for maintenance of bronchospasm
associated with COPD, chronic bronchitis,
emphysema

Contraindications
Hypersensitivity to atropine

Interactions
None

Dose
Adult   2 inhalations qid; not to exceed 12
inhalations/24 hours.

Forms
Metered dose inhaler with mouthpiece

Adverse Effects
Palpitations, nervousness, dizziness, headache,
nausea, GI discomfort, dry mouth, cough,
exacerbation of symptoms, blurred vision

**Special Nursing Considerations
and Patient Education**
- Offer hard, sugar-free candy to relieve dry mouth.
- Assess for palpitations.
- Teach patient to
  - avoid spraying in or around eyes.
  - not exceed prescribed dose to avoid
    overdosage.

Isosorbide Dinitrate

Brand Name
Isordil, Iso-Bid, Sorbide

Actions
Coronary vasodilator; relaxes vascular smooth muscle. Onset evident: PO 15–30 minutes; sublingual 2–5 minutes; sustained-release 30 minutes.

Uses
Angina pectoris

Contraindications
Sensitivity to hypotension. *Use with caution:* Anemia, glaucoma, hyperthyroidism, intracranial pressure, MI

Interactions
Alcohol, antihypertensives, sympathomimetics

Dose
Adult   5–30 mg tid–qid; sustained-release: 40 mg q6–12h

Forms
Chewable, sublingual, and sustained-release tablets; sustained-release capsules

Adverse Effects
Blurred vision, dizziness, flushing, nausea,
orthostatic hypotension, reflex tachycardia,
vascular headache, vertigo, vomiting

Special Nursing Considerations
and Patient Education
- Protect medication from heat and light.
- Store medication In original containers.
- When discontinued, decrease dosage gradually.
- Administer on empty stomach.
- Monitor vital signs.
- Be aware that
  - tolerance can develop.
- Teach patient to
  - notify physician if pain is not relieved by 3
    tablets after 30 minutes.
  - change position slowly to decrease
    hypotension.
  - eliminate smoking when using sublingual
    tablets.
  - not swallow sublingual tablets.
  - avoid stress as much as possible.
  - use caution in cold weather and during
    strenuous exercise because of potential
    orthostatic hypotension.
  - notify physician for blurred vision, rash.

Isoxsuprine HCl

Brand Name
Vasodilan

Actions
Cerebral or peripheral vasodilator; inhibits smooth uterine and vascular muscles. Onset evident in 1 hour.

Uses
Arteriosclerotic disease, Buerger's disease, cerebrovascular insufficiency, dysmenorrhea, peripheral vascular spasm, Raynaud's disease

Contraindications
Arterial hemorrhage, hypotension and tachycardia (parenteral forms), postpartum patients. *Use with caution:* Circulatory impairment of heart or brain, hypotension, tachycardia

Interactions
Tricyclic antidepressants

Dose
Adult　PO: 10–20 mg tid–qid; IM: 5–10 mg bid–tid

Forms
Injection, tablets

Adverse Effects
Dizziness, flushing, light-headedness, nausea, nervousness, palpitations, orthostatic hypotension, rash, vomiting

Special Nursing Considerations and Patient Education
- Monitor blood pressure, pulse; with threatened abortion, monitor duration, frequency, intensity of contractions.
- Discontinue for rash.
- Teach patient to
  - change position slowly to decrease hypotension.
  - be cautious when driving or involved in potentially hazardous tasks.
  - decrease smoking to enhance effectiveness of medication.

Ketoprofen

Brand Name
Orudis

Actions
Nonsteroidal anti-inflammatory. Onset evident:
analgesic 1–2 days; anti-inflammatory 3–7 days.

Uses
Acute or long-term treatment of rheumatoid
arthritis and osteoarthritis, mild-moderate pain,
primary dysmenorrhea

Contraindications
Hypersensitivity to aspirin, active GI bleeding,
active ulcers. *Use with caution:* history of GI
bleeding, cardiac disorders, ulcers, renal disease,
hepatic disease

Interactions
Aspirin, hydrochlorothiazide, probenecid, lithium,
methotrexate, phenobarbital, oral anticoagulants

Dose
Adult   PO: arthritis: initial dose: 75 mg tid or 50 mg
qid; *maintenance* dose: 150–300 mg in 3–4
divided doses; pain: 25–50 mg q6–8h prn;
maximum dose: 300 mg qd

Forms
Capsules

Adverse Effects
Dyspepsia, nausea, vomiting, abdominal pain,
diarrhea, flatulence, constipation, anorexia,
headache, dizziness, insomnia, dreams,
nervousness, rash, tinnitus, blood dyscrasias,
blurred vision

**Special Nursing Considerations
and Patient Education**
- Assess pain.
- Administer 30 minutes ac or 2 hours pc.
- Administer with food to decrease GI discomfort.
- Inform patient that therapeutic effects may take
  up to 1 month.
- Teach patient to
  - avoid aspirin and aspirin products.
  - remain in an upright position 15 minutes after
    taking medication.
  - avoid alcohol, driving.
  - take medication as prescribed; do not double
    dose.
  - notify physician if blurred vision or tinnitis occur.

Lebetalol

Brand Name
Normodyne, Trandate

Actions
Antihypertensive; non-selective beta blocker.
Onset evident: PO: 20 minutes–2 hours; IV 2–5
minutes.

Uses
Hypertension

Contraindications
Bronchial asthma, overt cardiac failure, greater
than first degree heart block, cardiogenic shock,
CHF, pulmonary edema, severe bradycardia. *Use
with caution:* impaired hepatic or renal function,
hypoglycemia

Interactions
Tricyclic antidepressants, cimetidine, nitroglycerin,
digoxin, halothane, beta-adrenergic bronchodilators, insulin, lidocaine

Dose
Adult   PO: initial dose: 100 mg bid; may increase q
2–3 days in increments of 100 mg bid;
maintenance dose: 200–400 mg bid; severe
hypertension: 1200–2400 mg/day; IV: 20 mg
over 2 minutes; may repeat 40–80 mg at 10-
minute intervals

Forms
Tablets, solution

Adverse Effects
Dizziness, fatigue, nausea, vomiting, dyspepsia, parathedias, nasal stuffiness, ejaculation failure, impotence, edema, weakness, hypotension, bradycardia, diarrhea, tinnitis, rash, abdominal pain, taste distortion

Special Nursing Considerations
and Patient Education
• Monitor blood pressure throughout treatment.
• Assess edema, I&O, weight.
• Taper withdrawal over 2 weeks; do not stop abruptly.
• Administer ac and hs.
• Assess for signs of CHF.
• IV—200 mg to 160 ml diluent (Lactated Ringers, solution with dextrose and saline).
• Do not dilute IV with sodium bicarbonate.
• Teach patient to
  – change position slowly.
  – not stop medication without physician's order.
  – be aware of signs of impending cardiac failure.
  – not use OTC medications, alcohol.
  – follow diet, exercise, stress reduction, weight loss program.

Levodopa

Brand Name
Larodopa, Sinemet

Actions
Changes into dopamine in CNS. Onset evident in 2–3 weeks.

Uses
Carbon monoxide or manganese poisoning, idiopathic or postencephalitic parkinsonism

Contraindications

Meds Adrenergics, MAO inhibitors

Other Blood dyscrasias, children under 12, history of melanoma, hypertension, narrow-angle glaucoma, suspicious skin lesions. *Use with caution:* Bronchial asthma; cardiovascular disease; convulsions; CVA; diabetes; dysrhythmias; emphysema; endocrine, hepatic, or renal disorders; history of MI; hypertension; neuroses; physiologic disorders with an organic base; psychoses; wide-angle glaucoma

Interactions
Amphetamines, anticholinergics, antihypertensives, antimuscarinics, ephedrine, guanethidine, haloperidol, hypoglycemics, MAO inhibitors, methyldopa, phenothiazines, phenylephrine, phenytoin, pyridoxine, reserpine, sympathomimetics, thioxanthenes, tranquilizers, vitamin B_6

Dose

Adult Initial dose: 0.5–1 gm/day in 2 or more doses with food; increase dose every 3–7 days as tolerated; usual therapeutic dose should not exceed 8 gm/day

Peds Over 12: same as Adult

Forms
Capsules, tablets

Adverse Effects
Adventitious, choreiform, or dystonic movements; akinesia; anorexia; anxiety; bruxism; constipation; depression; diarrhea; dysphagia; fatigue; grimacing; hypertension; insomnia; orthostatic hypotension; palpitations; weakness

**Special Nursing Considerations
and Patient Education**
- Protect medication from direct light.
- Monitor for behavior changes, indications of suicide ideation, vital signs.
- Teach patient
  – to not take vitamins that contain 10–25 mg of vitamin B_6.

  – to take with meals to decrease irritation.
  – to be cautious when driving or involved in potentially hazardous tasks.
  – to use caution during strenuous exercise if has a history of cardiac problems.
  – to change position slowly to decrease hypotension.
  – that medication may turn perspiration and/or urine pink or red.

Lisinopril

Brand Name
Prinvil, Zestril

Actions
Angiotensin-converting enzyme inhibitor,
antihypertensive

Uses
Hypertension—alone or with other
antihypertensives

Contraindications
Hypersensitivity. *Use with caution:* impaired renal
function, CHF

Interactions
Diuretics, indomethacin, potassium-sparing
diuretics, potassium-salt substitutes, potassium
supplements, antihypertensives.

Dose
Adult   PO: *initial dose*: 10 mg/day; *maintenance*
dose: 20–40 mg qd

Forms
Tablets

216

Adverse Effects

Dizziness, headache, fatigue, diarrhea, upper
respiratory problems, cough, nausea, orthostatic
effects, rash, asthenia, chest pain, vomiting,
dyspnea, proteinuria, urinary frequency,
angioedema

Special Nursing Considerations
and Patient Education

- Observe for signs of angioedema.
- Administer epinephrine as ordered for difficulty
  with breathing.
- Monitor blood pressure—lying and standing—q 4
  hours.
- Monitor electrolytes.
- Monitor I&O.
- Teach patient to
  - notify physician of signs and symptoms of
    angioedema (e.g., swelling of face, extremities,
    eyes, lips, tongue, difficulty in swallowing or
    breathing).
  - change position slowly.
  - not use salt substitutes without notifying
    physician.
  - avoid OTC medications.

Lithium Carbonate

Brand Name
Eskalith, Lithane, Lithobid, Lithonate, Lithotabs

Actions
Antimanic; alters neuronal characteristics. Onset evident in 1–3 weeks.

Uses
Psychoses (manic–depression)

Contraindications
Brain damage, cardiovascular dysfunction, children under 12, renal disease, pregnant women. *Use with caution:* CNS disorders, dehydration, diabetes, hypotension, hypothyroidism, low-sodium diet, renal insufficiency, severe infections, urinary retention

Interactions
Acetazolamide, aminophylline, chlorpromazine, diuretics, dyphylline, haloperidol, iodide preparations, mannitol, oxtriphylline, phenytoin, sodium bicarbonate, theophylline

Dose
Adult   Initial dose: 600 mg tid; *maintenance* dose: 300 mg tid–qid
Peds   Over 12: same as Adult

Forms
Capsules, sustained-release tablets, tablets

Adverse Effects
Diarrhea, dizziness, drowsiness, dry mouth,
extrapyramidal symptoms, headache, nausea,
pulse irregularities, tremors, vomiting

**Special Nursing Considerations
and Patient Education**
- Monitor fluid levels, lithium serum levels (effective
  range: 1-1.5 mEq; maintenance range: 0.6–1.2
  mEq), salt intake, weight.
- Arrange to have lithium levels drawn regularly
  (generally, daily until therapeutic dose
  established, then every 2 months).
- Be aware that
  - medication affects certain diagnostic tests (e.g.,
    serum enzymes, glucose, magnesium).
- Teach patient to
  - notify physician for decrease in coordination,
    diarrhea, hand tremors, lethargy, muscle
    weakness, slurring of speech, vomiting.
  - not take any nonprescription medications
    without notifying physician.
  - take medication with milk or food to decrease
    gastric upset.
  - be cautious when driving or involved in
    potentially hazardous tasks.
  - use caution in hot weather and during
    strenuous exercise because they decrease
    patient's tolerance to lithium.

Loperamide Hydrochloride

Brand Name
Imodium

Actions
Antidiarrheal. Onset evident in 1 hour.

Uses
Acute and chronic diarrhea, decrease volume of
ileostomy drainage

Contraindications
Hypersensitivity, acute dysentery, severe
ulcerative colitis, abdominal pain of unknown
origin

Interactions
None

Dose
Adult PO: initial dose: 4 mg, then 2 mg after each
unformed stool; *maximum* dose: 16 mg/day
Ped PO: 2–5 yr: 1 mg tid; 6–8 yr: 2 mg bid; 8–12
yr: 2 mg tid

Forms
Capsules

Adverse Effects
Rash, abdominal pain, nausea, vomiting,
constipation, tiredness, drowsiness, dizziness, dry
mouth

220

**Special Nursing Considerations
and Patient Education**
- Administer after each unformed stool.
- Provide adequate fluids, electrolyte replacement.
- Provide hard, sugar-free candy to relieve dry mouth.
- Monitor electrolytes if an long-term treatment.
- Assess skin for dehydration.
- Assess bowel sounds and stools prior to and during therapy.
- Teach patient to
  - notify physician if diarrhea does not stop after 48 hours.

Lorazepam

Brand Name
Ativan

Actions
Benzodiazepine, anti-anxiety, sedative/hypnotic.
Onset evident: PO 15–45 minutes; IM 15–30
minutes; IV 5–15 minutes.

Uses
Anxiety disorders, short-term relief of symptoms
of anxiety or anxiety associated with depression,
preanesthesia

Contraindications
Hypersensitivity, acute narrow-angle glaucoma,
comatose patients, preexisting CNS depression,
psychosis. *Use with caution:* elderly or debilitated
patients, hepatic or renal disease, suicidal
patients, patients who abuse substances

Interactions
Alcohol, antihistamines, narcotics,
antidepressants, oral contraceptives, valproic
acid, MAO inhibitors, tricyclic antidepressants,
scopolamine, cigarettes, levodopa

Dose
Adult   PO: 2–6 mg/day in divided doses; *maximum*
dose: 10 mg/day; IM: 0.05 mg/kg (not to
exceed 4 mg) 2 hours preop; IV: 0.044 mg/
kg (not to exceed 2 mg) 15–20 minutes
preop

Forms
  Tablets, IM & IV injection

Adverse Effects
  Sedation, depression, fatigue, dizziness,
  drowsiness, lethargy, paradoxical excitation,
  orthostatic hypotension, blurred vision,
  extrapyrimidal symptoms, dry mouth, changes in
  libido, nasal congestion

**Special Nursing Considerations
and Patient Education**
- Administer largest dose at hs.
- Provide safety measures.
- Administer IM deeply.
- Offer hard, sugar-free candy to relieve dry mouth.
- Administer IV at rate of 2 mg over a 1-minute
  period.
- Do not administer intra-arterially.
- Do not use solutions that are discolored or have
  precipitate.
- Teach patient to
  - notify physician of suspected pregnancy.
  - change position slowly.
  - take as directed; do not double the dose.
  - avoid driving.
  - avoid alcohol.

Lovasitatin

Brand Name
Mevacor

Actions
Antihyperlipidemic. Onset evident within 2 weeks; peaks in 2–4 hours.

Uses
Adjunct to diet for reduction of elevated and total LDL cholesterol levels in patient with primary hypercholesterolemia, mixed hyperlipidemia

Contraindications
Hypersensitivity, pregnancy, lactation, liver dysfunction. *Use with caution:* alcoholics, past liver diseases, hypotension, severe acute infections, uncontrolled seizure disorders, electrolyte imbalances

Interactions
Bile acid sequestrants, coumadin, cyclosporine, gemfibrozil, niacin

Dose
Adult   PO: 20 mg qd with evening meal to start; may increase 20–80 mg/day in single or divided doses; adjust dose every month

Forms
   Tablets

Adverse Effects
   Constipation, diarrhea, dyspepsia, flatus,
   abdominal discomfort, nausea, rash, myalgia,
   headache, dizziness, heartburn, fatigue, insomnia

**Special Nursing Considerations
and Patient Education**
- Store in light-resistant container.
- Administer in evening.
- Arrange for low-cholesterol diet; refer to diet.
- Assess cholesterol levels periodically during
  therapy.
- Arrange liver function studies every 1–2 months.
- Teach patient to
  - have periodic opthalmologic examinations.
  - take medication in evening.
  - follow diet and exercise therapy.

Loxapine Succinate

Brand Name
Loxitane

Actions
Antipsychotic, tranquilizer. Onset evident in 20–30 minutes.

Uses
Psychotic disorders, schizophrenia

Contraindications
Meds   Alcohol, CNS depressants
Other   Children under 16, coma. *Use with caution:* Brain tumor, cardiovascular dysfunction, convulsive disorders, glaucoma, hypertension, hypotension, intestinal obstruction, syncope, tachycardia, urinary retention

Interactions
Anticholinergics, guanethidine

Dose
Adult   PO: Initial dose: 10 mg bid; *maintenance* dose: 60–100 mg bid–qid; *maximum* dose: 250 mg/day

Forms
Capsules, concentrate, injection

Adverse Effects
Blurred vision, constipation, drowsiness, dry
mouth, extrapyramidal symptoms, orthostatic
hypotension, photosensivity

**Special Nursing Considerations
and Patient Education**
• Dilute concentrate with water or juice (e.g.,
  grapefruit, orange).
• Monitor for fine vermicular tongue movements
  (may indicate early tardive dyskinesia).
• Offer hard candy (regular or sugar-free) to relieve
  dry mouth.
• Teach patient
  – to be cautious when driving or involved in
    potentially hazardous tasks.
  – that medication may cause photosensitivity.
  – to notify physician for blurred vision, tremors,
    weakness.
  – to change position slowly.
  – to use sunscreen.

Medroxyprogesterone Acetate

Brand Name
Amen, Curretab, Provera

Actions
Hormanal agent, antineoplastic

Uses
Secondary amenorrhea, abnormal uterine
bleeding, renal carcinoma, endometrial carcinoma

Contraindications
Thrombophlebitis, thromboembolic disorders, liver
disease, genital bleeding or carcinoma, breast
carcinoma, hypersensitivity. *Use with caution:*
depression, hypertension, lactation, blood
dyscrasias, migraines, renal disease, family
history of breast carcinoma or reproductive tract
carcinoma.

Interactions
Bromocryptine

Dose
Adult PO: secondary amenorrhea: 5–10 mg qd ×
5–10 days; start treatment at any time in the
menustral cycle; uterine bleeding: 5–10 mg
qd × 5–10 days; begin on 16th day of cycle;
IM: carcinoma: 400–1000 mg/ week

Forms
Tablets, injection

Adverse Effects
Dizziness, breakthrough bleeding, spottings
change in flow, edema, amenorrhea, weight
change, cervical changes, cholestatic jaundice,
rash, depression, pyrexia, insomnia, nausea,
fatigue, migraines, myocardial infarction,
thromboembolism, CVA, pulmonary embolism,
diplopia, gynecomastial impotence, spontaneous
abortion, hyperglycemia, photosensitivity

**Special Nursing Considerations
and Patient Education**
- Administer with food or milk to decrease GI
  symptoms.
- Administer IM deeply; rotate sites.
- Store in dark container.
- Assess mental status.
- Teach patient to
  - utilize sunscreen.
  - report suspected pregnancy.
  - report breast lumps, vaginal bleeding, chest
    pain, leg pain, edema.

Meperidine HCl

Brand Name
  Demerol

Actions
  Antispasmodic, CNS depressant (cortical,
  subcortical levels), narcotic analgesic. Onset
  evident in 15 minutes.

Uses
  Preoperative medication, severe pain

Contraindications
Meds   Alcohol, MAO Inhibitors
Other Gallbladder or bile duct disorders, hepatic
         dysfunction, increased intracranial pressure.
         Use with caution: Addison's disease, cardiac
         dysrhythmias, epilepsy, glaucoma, head
         injuries, hypothyroidism, prostatic
         hypertrophy, renal dysfunction, respiratory
         impairment, urethral stricture

Interactions
  Anticholinergics, antidepressants, CNS
  depressants, diuretics, hypnotics, narcotics,
  sedatives, skeletal muscle relaxants, tranquilizers

Dose
Adult PO: 50–150 mg q3–4h
Peds   PO: 1 mg/kg q4h prn

Forms
Injection, tablets

Adverse Effects
Dizziness, dry mouth, euphoria, headache, lightheadedness, nausea, orthostatic hypotension, respiratory difficulty, syncope, tachycardia, vomiting

Special Nursing Considerations and Patient Education
- Check blood pressure and respiratory rate prior to administration. Respirations should be at least 12/minute; BP per individual guidelines. Hold dose if minimum levels are not met.
- Offer hard candy (regular or sugar-free) to relieve dry mouth.
- Rotate injection sites.
- Monitor level of pain prior to and during administration.
- Be aware that dependence and tolerance are possible.
- Administer with food to decrease GI discomfort.
- Teach patient to
  - avoid alcohol and other CNS depressants.
  - be cautious when driving or involved in potentially hazardous tasks.
  - not smoke after receiving medications because of safety factor.
  - change position slowly to decrease hypotension.

Meprobamate

Brand Name
Equanil, Meprospan, Miltown

Actions
Antianxiety, anticonvulsant, hypnotic, muscle relaxant, sedative. Onset evident in less than 1 hour.

Uses
Anxiety, insomnia, tension

Contraindications
Meds Alcohol, CNS depressants
Other Acute Intermittent porphyria, allergy to chemically related medications, children under 6 years. *Use with caution:* Epilepsy, hepatic or renal dysfunction

Interactions
Anticonvulsants, antidepressants, hypnotics, MAO inhibitors, oral anticoagulants, sedatives, tranquilizers

Dose
Adult PO: 400 mg tid-qid; *maximum* dose: 2.4 gm/day
Peds PO: Over 6 yr: initial dose, 100–200 mg bid-tid

Forms
Injection, suspension, sustained-release capsules, tablets

Adverse Effects
Blurred vision, dizziness, drowsiness, dysrhythmias, hypotension, paresthesia, slurring of speech, syncope, weakness

**Special Nursing Considerations
and Patient Education**
- Do not crush sustained-release capsules.
- Use caution when administering to a patient with suicidal potential; ensure patient swallows dose.
- Help patient to verbalize anxious feelings.
- Discontinue for ecchymosis, fever, hemorrhage, rash, sore throat.
- Be aware that
  - dependence is possible; when discontinued, decrease dosage gradually.
- Teach patient
  - to be cautious when driving or involved in potentially hazardous tasks.
  - to change position slowly since dizziness from hypotension may result in injury.
  - to decrease caffeine intake because of its stimulant effect.
  - to notify physician of suspected pregnancy.

Metaproterenol

Brand Name
Alupent, Metaprel

Actions
Bronchodilator. Onset evident: PO 15 minutes;
Inhaler 1–5 minutes.

Uses
Bronchial asthma, reversible bronchospasm that
occurs with bronchitis and emphysema

Contraindications
Hypersensitivity, narrow-angle glaucoma. *Use
with caution:* hypertension, coronary artery
disease, CHF, hyperthyroidism, diabetes mellitus.
cardiac disorders, psychonourosis, history of
seizures, CVA

Interactions
MAO inhibitors, beta blockers, sympathomimetics,
halothane, cyclopropane, insulin, oral hypoglycemics

Dose
Adult   PO: 20 mg tid/qid; inhalation: 2–3 inhalations
q 3–4 h; not to exceed 12 inhalations/day
Peds   PO: under 9 yr and 27kg: 1 tsp tid/qid over 9
yrs and 27kg: 2 tsp tid/qid; 6–9 yrs: 10 mg
tid/qid; over 9 yr: 20 mg tid/qid

Forms
Inhalation aerosol, tablets, syrup

Adverse Effects
Nervousness, tachycardia, tremor, hypertension,
restlessness, anxiety, drowsiness, irritability,
weakness, vertigo, insomnia, palpitations, change
in blood pressure, nausea, vomiting, dyspnea

**Special Nursing Considerations
and Patient Education**
- Administer with food to decrease GI discomfort.
- Instruct patient in proper usage of inhaler.
- Wait 1–2 minutes between inhalations.
- Administer 2 hours before hs.
- Teach patient to
    - use for minimal amount of time.
    - not exceed recommended dosage.
    - avoid OTC medications.
    - inform physician if side effects occur.
    - avoid smoking.

Methohexital Sodium

Brand Name
Brevital

Actions
Anesthetic

Uses
Hypnotic induction, surgery

Contraindications
Meds   Alcohol, CNS depressants
Other Status asthmaticus, porphyria. *Use with
          caution:* Addison's disease, anemia,
          cardiovascular disease, hepatic or renal
          dysfunction, hypertension, increased
          intracranial pressure or serum urea,
          myasthenia gravis, myxedema

Interactions
Acid solutions

Dose
Adult   Individualized; initial dose: 50–120 mg IV;
          maintenance dose: 20–40 mg q4–7min

Forms
Injection

236

Adverse Effects

Abnormal muscle movements, bronchospasm, dysrhythmias, hiccoughs, laryngospasm, myocardial or respiratory depression, sneezing

Special Nursing Considerations and Patient Education

- Maintain a patent airway.
- Do not mix any other medications in infusion solution.
- Do not use bacteriostatic diluents.
- Monitor vital signs every q 3–5 minutes.
- Keep endotracheal intubation, resuscitation equipment, and oxygen readily available.

Methyldopa

Brand Name
Aldomet

Actions
Stimulates alpha-adrenergic receptors (central Inhibiting). Onset evident: PO 6–12 hours; IV 4–6 hours.

Uses
Complicated, renal hypertension; hypertension

Contraindications
Meds Alcohol, CNS depressants, MAO Inhibitors, tricyclic antidepressants
Other History of depression, pheochromocytoma. *Use with caution:* Bilateral cerebrovascular disease, history of hepatic disease, renal impairment

Interactions
Amphetamines, antihypertensives, haloperidol

Dose
Adult PO: 250 mg bid-tid ×3/day; *maintenance* dose: 500 mg–2 gm/day in divided doses
Peds PO: 10–65 mg/kg/day in 2–4 divided doses

Forms
Injection (-pate hydrochloride), tablets

Adverse Effects
  Bradycardia, depression, diarrhea, dizziness,
  edema, headache, hepatitis, nausea, orthostatic
  hypotension, positive direct Coombs' test,
  sedation, vomiting, weakness

Special Nursing Considerations
and Patient Education
- Adjust dosage at 2-day intervals in order to reach
  a maintenance dosage.
- When changing medication to or from other
  antihypertensives, do so gradually.
- Monitor blood pressure, I&O, neurologic status,
  renal function, weight.
- Be aware that
  - tolerance can develop if patient is not on a
    diuretic.
- Teach patient
  - that hot baths or showers may aggravate
    hypotension.
  - to change position slowly to decrease
    hypotension.
  - that medication may cause tongue to appear
    black or turn urine blue/dark.
  - that medication may cause photosensitivity.
  - to be cautious when driving or involved in
    potentially hazardous tasks.
  - to use caution during strenuous exercise as it
    may increase orthostatic hypotension.
  - to notify physician for fever, urine darkening.

Methylphenidate HCl

Brand Name
Ritalin Hydrochloride

Actions
CNS stimulant; affects the cerebral cortex and subcortical structures

Uses
Attention-deficit disorders, hyperkinesis, mild depression, narcolepsy, withdrawn senile behavior

Contraindications
Meds MAO Inhibitors, pressors
Other Agitation, anxiety, children under 6, glaucoma, severe depression, tension. *Use with caution:* Emotional instability, epilepsy, history of alcoholism or drug dependence, hypertension, psychosis

Interactions
Anticholinergics, anticoagulants, anticonvulsants, desipramine, guanethidine, imipramine, phenobarbital, phenytoin, primadone, tricyclic antidepressants

Dose
Adult PO: 20–30 mg/day in 2–3 divided doses
Peds PO: 5 mg before breakfast or lunch; increased by 5–10 mg weekly; *maximum* dose: 60 mg/day

240

Forms
   Injection, tablets

Adverse Effects
   Angina, anorexia, blurred vision, dizziness,
   dyskinesia, headache, insomnia, nervousness,
   tachycardia, weight loss

**Special Nursing Considerations
and Patient Education**
* Administer medication 30–45 minutes before
   meals.
* Monitor blood pressure, pulse, weight.
* In children, discontinue if there is no evidence of
   improvement within one month; long-term therapy
   may impair growth.
* If patient has insomnia, administer last dose by
   6:00 P.M.
* Be aware that
   – dependence is possible; when discontinued,
      gradually decrease dosage.
   – tolerance can develop.
* Teach patient
   – to be cautious when driving or involved in
      potentially hazardous tasks.
   – to monitor weight; report loss to physician.
   – to avoid alcohol, caffeine.

Metoclopramide Hydrochloride

Brand Name
Reglan

Actions
Antiemetic, dopaminergic-blocking agent, GI stimulant. Onset evident: PO 30–60 minutes; IM 10–15 minutes; IV 1–3 minutes.

Uses
Prevention of postoperative nausea and vomiting, nausea and vomiting caused by chemotherapy and gastroesophageal reflux, small bowel intubation, radiological examination

Contraindications
GI obstruction, pheochromocytoma, history of seizures

Interactions
CNS depressants, alcohol, insulin, haloperidol, phenothiazines, sedatives

Dose
Adult   IV: antiemetic: 1–2 mg/kg q2–3h ×3–5 days; IV: facilitate intubation and examination: 10 mg; gastric statis: 10 mg 30 minutes ac, hs
Peds   IV: facilitate intubation and examination: 6–14 yr: 2.5–5 mg; under 6 yr: 0.1 mg/ kg

Forms
Tablets, injection, syrup

Adverse Efffects
Drowsiness, fatigue, extrapyramidal reactions, restlessness, nausea, diarrhea, headache, sleeplessness, dry mouth, transient flushing of face and upper body (IV)

**Special Nursing Considerations
and Patient Education**
- Assess bowel sounds, abdominal distention.
- Assess for extrapyramidal reactions.
- Administer 30 minutes ac.
- Administer IV over 1–2 minutes.
- Diluted IV solution is stable for 24–48 hours.
- Provide emotional support of diagnosis.
- Teach patient to
  - avoid driving until stabilized.
  - avoid alcohol, OTC medications, CNS depressants.
  - notify physician if signs of extrapyramidal reactions occur.

Metoprolol Tartrate

Brand Name
Lopressor

Actions
Antihypertensive; stops access of catecholamine
to neurotransmitters to cardiac muscle beta, receptors. Onset evident: PO 10 minutes.

Uses
Hypertension

Contraindications
Meds MAO inhibitors
Other Cardiogenic shock, children, overt cardiac
failure, sinus bradycardia. *Use with caution:*
Angina, bronchospastic disease, cardiac
dysfunction, congestive heart failure,
diabetes, hepatic or renal impairment,
thyrotoxicosis

Interactions
Digitalis, diuretics, dobutamine, dopamine,
isoproterenol, norepinephrine bitartrate, reserpine

Dose
Adult Individualized; initial dose: 50 mg bid
adjusted weekly; *maintenance* dose: 100 mg
bid

Forms
Tablets

Adverse Effects
Bradycardia, congestive heart failure, constipation, depression, diarrhea, disorientation, dizziness, dyspepsia, fatigue, hallucinations, hypotension, nausea, palpitations, shortness of breath, wheezing

Special Nursing Considerations and Patient Education
- Administer medication before meals to enhance absorption.
- Monitor blood pressure, neurologic status, renal function, I&O.
- Teach patient to
  - be cautious when driving or involved in potentially hazardous tasks.
  - not discontinue without notifying physician.
  - follow additional hypertensive regime: weight loss, low-sodium diet, stress management.

Metronidazole

Brand Name
  Flagyl

Actions
  Amebicide, antiprotozoan, systemic trichomonacide; hinders release of hydrogen for metabolic use in susceptible microorganisms

Uses
  Chagas disease, giardiasis, hepatic or luminal form of *Entamoeba histolytica,* leishmaniasis

Contraindications
Meds Alcohol
Other Blood dyscrasias, CNS organic disease. *Use with caution:* Diabetes

Interactions
  Oral anticoagulants

Dose
Adult PO: 250 mg tid × 7 days; IV: 15 mg/kg over 1 hr (load), then 7.5 mg/kg q6h
Peds PO: 35–50 mg/kg/day in 3 divided doses ×10 days

Forms
  Injection, tablets

Adverse Effects

Abdominal cramps, anorexia, ataxia, constipation, diarrhea, dry mouth, headache, metallic taste, nausea, paresthesia, rash, seizures, vomiting

Special Nursing Considerations and Patient Education

- Protect medication from light.
- Arrange treatment for sexual partner(s).
- Offer hard candy (regular or sugar-free) to relieve dry mouth.
- Teach patient
  - that medication may cause a metallic taste in mouth or dark brown urine.
  - to be cautious when driving or involved in
  - potentially hazardous tasks.
  - to notify physician if numbness in feet and/or hands occurs.
  - take with food.
  - to take as prescribed.

Miconazole Nitrate

Brand Name
  Monistat, Monistat IV

Actions
  Antifungal. Onset: IV rapid.

Uses
  Severe systemic fungal infections, fungal urinary
  bladder infections, moniliasis, tinea palis, tinea
  cruris. IV is used for severe infections.

Contraindications
  Hypersensitivity, renal disease, hepatic disease.
  Do not use vaginal medication with diaphragm in
  place

Interactions
  Warfarin, anticoagulants, amphotericin

Dose
Adult IV: 200–3600 mg/day divided in doses q8h;
  topical: apply to area bid; vaginal: apply qhs
  for 1 week; bladder infection: 200 mg q6–12h
Peds IV: 20–40mg/kg/day; *maximum dose:* 15
  mg/kg/day

Forms
  Injection-IV, aerosol, cream, lotion, powder
  vaginal cream, vaginal suppositories

Adverse Effects
Phlebitis, rash, nausea and vomiting, febrile reactions, hypedemia, increased libido, itching, valvovaginal burning, alleric contact dermatitis

Special Nursing Considerations and Patient Education
- Avoid rapid IV infusion.
- Insert vaginal suppository high in vagina, with the patient remaining recumbent for 10 minutes.
- Provide sanitary pad.
- Discard prepared IV solution after 24 hours.
- Do not use occlusive dressings.
- Apply topical using gloves.
- Teach patient to
  - utilize full length of treatment.
  - utilize good hygiene to decrease reinfection. continue during menstrual period.
  - refrain from intercourse (vaginal) or have partner use condom.
  - notify physician if burning, pain, or rash occur.

Morphine Sulfate

Brand Name
Morphine

Actions
Analgesic; impedes pain impulses at subcortical level. Onset evident in 20 minutes.

Uses
Burns, pain, shock

Contraindications
Alcohol, CNS depressants. *Use with caution:* Acute alcoholism, Addison's disease, atrial flutter, cardiac dysrhythmias, convulsive disorders, gallbladder disease, head injuries, hepatic or renal dysfunction, hypotension, hypothyroidism, myxedema , prostatic hypertrophy, toxic psychosis

Interactions
Anesthetics, anticholinergics, antihistamines, benzodiazepines, MAO inhibitors, papaverine, phenothiazines, skeletal muscle relaxants, tricyclic antidepressants

Dose
Adult   PO: 5–15 mg q4h
Peds   PO: 0.1–0.2 mg/kg/dose; *maximum* dose: 15 mg/single dose

Forms
Atropine injection, injection, tablets

Adverse Effects
Anorexia, constipation, drowsiness, dysphoria, euphoria, hypotension, nausea, respiratory depression, spasm of biliary tract, tremors, vomiting, weakness

Special Nursing Considerations and Patient Education
- Protect medication from direct light.
- If respirations are less than 10–12, hold medication.
- When discontinued, decrease dose gradually.
- Monitor bowel pattern, I&O, vital signs.
- Be aware that
  – patient may become addicted to medication.
- Teach (hospital) patient to
  – not smoke or walk without assistance due to the presence of possible side effects.
  – change position slowly to decrease hypotension.
  – take with food.

Nadolol

Brand Name
Corganol, Corgard

Actions
Antihypertensive, antiangina. Onset evident within 5 days.

Uses
Hypertension, angina pectoris

Contraindications
Bronchial asthma, sinus bradycardia, cardiogenic shock, overt cardiac failure, secondary or tertiary degree heart block, bronchospastic disease, COPD. *Use with caution:* hypoglycemia

Interactions
Digoxin, halothane, captopril, cimetidine, chlorapromazine, oral contraceptives, thyroid hormones, Norepinephrine, dopamine, insulin, succinylcholine, clonidine, theophylline, calcium channel blockers, phenobarbital

Dose
Adult   PO: angina: initial dose: 40 mg qd; may increase (every 3–7 days) to 40–80 mg qd; hypertension: initial dose: 40 mg qd; may increase to 80–320 mg qd

Forms
Tablets

Adverse Effects
Bradycardia, dizziness, fatigue, sedation, nausea,
vomiting, diarrhea, abdominal discomfort,
anorexia, rash, headache, dry mouth,
hypotension, cramps, vertigo, flatulence,
weakness

**Special Nursing Considerations
and Patient Education**
- Monitor vital signs, blood pressure.
- Provide safety measures.
- Monitor I&O.
- Notify physician if pulse is less than 50.
- Observe for signs of CHF.
- Teach patient to
  - change position slowly.
  - not take OTC medications.
  - avoid driving.
  - not discontinue medication abruptly.
  - notify physician if pulse is less than 50.

Naloxone Hydrochloride

Brand Name
Narcan

Actions
Narcotic antagonist for receptor sites in CNS.
Onset evident in 2 minutes (IV).

Uses
Narcotic or respiratory depression, opiate
overdosage

Contraindications
Hypersensitivity

Interactions
None

Dose
Adult   0.4 mg/dose q2–3min; may have 2–3 doses
Peds   0.01 mg/kg/dose q2–3min; may have 2–3
          doses

Forms
Injection

Adverse Effects
Drowsiness, hypertension, hyperventilation,
nausea, tachycardia, tremors, vomiting

**Special Nursing Considerations
and Patient Education**
- Protect medication from direct light.
- Monitor vital signs.
- Monitor for signs of narcotic withdrawal:
  abdominal cramps, increased BP & temperature,
  vomiting.
- Be aware that
  - dependence is possible; when discontinued,
  - decrease dosage gradually.
  - failure of the patient to respond may indicate
  - that the respiratory depression is not only a
  - result from opiate intoxication.

Naproxen

Brand Name
Anaprox, Naprosyn

Actions
Non-narcotic analgesic, anti-inflammatory, antipyretic. Onset evident: analgesic 1 hour; anti-inflammatory 14 days.

Uses
Mild-moderate pain, primary dysmenorrhea, rheumatoid arthritis, osteoarthritis, juvenile arthritis, ankylosing spondylitis, tendinitis, bursitis, acute gout

Contraindications
Hypersensitivity, aspirin or other nonsteroidal anti-inflammatory medications that induce asthma, rhinitis and nasal polyps, GI bleeding, active peptic ulcer

Interactions
Heparin, hydantoin, sulfonamide, sulfonylurea, aspirin, lithium

Dose
Adult PO: pain: initial dose: 550 mg, then 275 mg q6–8h; *maximum* dose: 1,375 mg/day; arthritis: 275–550 mg bid; gout: initial dose: 825 mg then 275 mg q8h

Peds PO: arthritis: 10 mg/kg/day in 2 divided doses

Forms
Tablets, suspension

Adverse Effects
Constipation, heartburn, abdominal pain, nausea, headache, dizziness, drowsiness, pruritis, skin eruptions, ecchymoses, tinnitus, edema, dyspnea

**Special Nursing Considerations
and Patient Education**
- Assess blood, renal and liver status prior to and during therapy.
- Administer on empty stomach if possible.
- Inform patient that therapeutic effects may take up to 4 weeks.
- Assess pain prior to and during therapy.
- Assess for asthma, rhinitis, urticaria.
- Teach patient to
  - be aware of drowsiness and dizziness while driving.
  - avoid alcohol and OTC medications.
  - notify physician if rash, asthma, rhinitis or visual distubances occur.

Naproxen (Sodium)

Brand Name
Naprosyn, Anaprox

Actions
Non-narcotic analgesics nonsteroidal anti-inflammatory. Onset evident: analgesic 1 hour; anti-inflammatory 14 days.

Uses
Mild-moderate pain, primary dysmenorrhea, rheumatoid arthritis, osteoarthritis, juvenile arthritis, tendinitis, bursitis, acute gout

Contraindications
Hypersensitivity, severe renal disease. *Use with caution:* ulcer disease, renal and hepatic disease

Interactions
Aspirin

Dose
Adult PO: pain and dysmenorrhea: initial dose: 500 mg, then 250 mg q6–8h; *maximum* dose: 1250 mg/day; inflammation: 250–275 mg bid
Peds PO: inflammation: 10 mg/kg/day in divided doses

258

Forms
Tablets

Adverse Effects
Headache, dizziness, drowsiness, nausea,
constipation, dypepsia, GI bleeding, abdominal
pain, heartburn, itching

**Special Nursing Considerations
and Patient Education**
* Assess pain—both degree and location—prior to
  administration and after peak of onset.
* Determine if the patient is allergic to aspirin, or
  has renal or hepatic disease.
* Administer initial dose 30 minutes before or 2
  hours after meals.
* Administer with food or milk to decrease GI
  discomfort (food slows absorption only).
* Teach patient to
  – Avoid OTC medications.

Nicotine Resin Complex

Brand Name
Nicorette

Actions
Smoking deterrent.

Uses
Deter cigarette smoking—temporary aid. Onset
evident in 15–30 minutes.

Contraindications
Non–smokers, immediate post–myocardial
infarction period, life-threatening arrhythmias,
severe or worsening angina pectoris, active
temporomandibular joint disease, pregnancy. *Use
with caution:* hypertension, peptic ulcer, diabetes
mellitus, oral or pharyngeal inflammation, history
of esophagitis, children

Interactions
Adrenergic agonists, adrenergic blockers,
caffeine, theophylline, phenacetin, imipramine,
pentazocine, cortisol, catacholamines

Dose
Adult   1 piece of gum when urge to smoke occurs;
not to exceed 30 pieces/day. Do not use
longer than 6 months.

Forms

2 mg square chewing piece

Adverse Effects

Excess salivation, dizziness, GI discomfort,
eructation, nausea, vomiting, mouth or throat
soreness, jaw muscle ache, hiccoughs, anorexia

**Special Nursing Considerations
and Patient Education**

- Instruct patient to stop smoking immediately.
- Schedule follow-up visits every 3–4 weeks.
- Instruct patient to chew gum slowly and
  intermittently.
- Taper use of medication after 3 months.
- Offer emotional support, behavior modification,
  encouragement.
- Teach patient to
  - not chew rapidly.
  - not exceed 30 pieces/day.
  - not chew each piece for more than 45 minutes.
  - not use during pregnancy.

Nifedipine

Brand Name
Procardea

Actions
Antihypetensive, antianginal, calcium channel blocker. Onset evident in 20 minutes.

Uses
Chronic stable angina, angina pectoris due to coronary vasospasm (Prinzmetal's Variant Angina), hypertension, Raynaud's Syndrome

Contraindications
Hypersensitivity. *Use with caution*: sick sinus syndrome, severe hepatic disease, congestive heart failure, aortic stenosis

Interactions
Beta-adrenergic blocking agents, digitalis, coumarin anticoagulants, cimetidine

Dose
Adult   PO: initial dose: 10 mg tid; *maintenance* dose: 10–20 mg tid; *maximum* dose: 180 mg/day

Forms
Tablets

Adverse Effects
Dizziness, lightheadedness, flushing, heat
sensation, headache, edema, nausea, rash,
heartburn, dysrhythmia, nasal congestion, cough,
wheeze

**Special Nursing Considerations
and Patient Education**
- Monitor I&O and weight daily.
- Observe for signs and symptoms of digitalis
  toxicity if on concurrent digitalis therapy.
- Administer with meals to decrease GI discomfort.
- Monitor vital signs and blood pressure.
- Teach patient to
  - change position slowly.
  - avoid driving if dizziness occurs.
  - decrease caffeine intake.

Nitrofurantoin Macrocrystals

Brand Name
Macrodantin

Actions
Anti-infective, antibacterial. Onset evident: PO 30 minutes; IV rapid.

Uses
Urinary tract infections due to E. coli, enterococci, S. aureus

Contraindications
Hypersensitivity, anuria, oliguria, several renal impairment

Interactions
Antacids, probenecid, magnesium trisilicate

Dose
Adult   PO: 50–100 mg qid; IV: 180 mg bid
Peds   PO: 5–7 mg/kg/24 hours

Forms
Capsules, solution

Adverse Effects
Chronic, subacute or acute pulmonary hypersensitivity (e.g. malaise, dyspnea on exertion, cough, fever, chills, chest pain), nausea, emesis, anorexia, photosensitivity, blood dyscrasias, exfoliative dermatitis

**Special Nursing Considerations
and Patient Education**

- Discontinue immediately if acute, subacute or chronic pulmonary reactions occur.
- Monitor CBC if on long-term therapy.
- Administer with food or milk.
- IV: prepare immediately prior to use; do not use alcohol swabs on vials; administer 50–60 gtt/min.
- Teach signs of pulmonary reaction.
- Monitor urine C & S.
- Teach patient to
  - rinse mouth after oral suspension to avoid tooth stains.
  - take as directed.
  - be aware that urine discoloration may occur.
  - notify physician if signs of pulmonary reaction occur.

Nitroglycerin

Brand Name
Nitro-Bid, Nitrol, Nitrostat

Actions
Vasodilator; relaxation of vascular smooth
muscle. Onset evident In 1–5 minutes.

Uses
Angina pectoris

Contraindications
Meds Alcohol
Other Anemia, children, glaucoma, hypersensitivity
to vasodilators, hyperthyroid, increased
intracranial pressure, MI, tendency to
hypotension

Interactions
Antihypertensives

Dose
Adult Individualized; PO: 2.5–6.5 mg q8–12h;
sublingual: 0.4–0.6 mg prn; IV: 5–20 mcg/
min

Forms
Injection, ointment, prolonged-action and
sublingual tablets, sustained-release capsules,
transdermal patch

Adverse Effects
Dizziness, flushing, headache, nausea, palpitations, postural hypotension, tachycardia, vomiting

Special Nursing Considerations and Patient Education
- Do not crush prolonged-action or sustained-release forms.
- When applying ointment, do not rub; rotate sites.
- When discontinued, decrease dosage and frequency over 4–6 weeks.
- Repeat dose if pain is not relieved in 5–10 minutes; consult physician if pain is not relieved in 15–20 minutes.
- Keep medication in original container; do not store with cotton.
- Do not use medication if it is older than 60 days.
- Be aware that
  - tolerance can develop.
  - medication is unstable; protect from air, heat, light, moisture.
- Teach patient to
  - change position slowly to decrease hypotension.
  - decrease smoking; be cautious in cold weather, during strenuous exercise, or with increased stress because these may cause increased episodes of angina pectoris.
  - not swallow sublingual tablets.
  - notify physician if blurred vision or dry mouth occurs.
  - keep sublingual tablets in original container; do not expose to air, moisture, heat.

Norfloxacin

Brand Name
Noroxin

Actions
Antibacterial; urinary tract anti-infective. Onset evident in 3–4 weeks.

Uses
Adults with urinary tract infections caused by susceptible gram-negative bacteria (e.g., E. coli, Proteus mirabilis)

Contraindications
Hypersensitivity, quinolone group of antibacterials. *Use with caution:* renal dysfunction, seizure disorders.

Interactions
Probenecid, nitrofurantoin, antacids

Dose
Adult   PO: uncomplicated UTI: 400 mg bid × 7–10 days; complicated UTI: 400 mg bid ×10–21 days

Forms
Tablets

Adverse Effects
Nausea, headache, dizziness, fatigue, rash,
abdominal pain, insomnia, dyspepsia, flatulence,
heartburn, constipation, diarrhea, dry mouth

Special Nursing Considerations
and Patient Education
- Store in tightly covered containers.
- Increase fluid intake.
- Administer 1 hour ac or 2 hour pc with water.
- Monitor I&O, urine pH.
- Assess urine culture and sensitivity.
- Teach patient to
  - take full prescribed amount.
  - avoid antacids within 2 hours of administration.

Nortriptyline Hydrochloride

Brand Name
Aventyl, Pamelor

Actions
Tricyclic antidepressant; interferes with transport, release and storage of catecholamines. Onset evident in 4–19 days.

Uses
Endogenous depression

Contraindications
Alcohol, MAO inhibitors, dibenzazepines, recovery period of MI, convulsive disorders. *Use with caution:* ECT, pre-existing cardiovascular disorders, narrow-angle glaucoma, suicidal patients, hyperthyroidism, impaired renal or hepatic function, schizophrenia, manic-depressives, elective surgery

Interactions
Cimetidine, phenothiazines, oral contraceptives, MAO inhibitors, thyroid medications, epinephrine, alcohol, barbiturates, CNS depressants, quinidine, nicotine, dicumarol, ephedrine

Dose
Adult PO: 25 mg tid/qid; may be given as a single dose; *maximum* dose: 150 mg/day
Peds (over 12yr) PO: 30–50 mg in divided doses

270

Forms
Capsules, liquid

Adverse Effects
Dizziness, drowsiness, confusion, headache,
anxiety, tremors, insomnia, constipation, dry
mouth, retention, orthostatic hypotension,
tachycardia, blurred vision, tinnitus, disorientation,
weakness, nausea, vomiting, weight changes,
sweating, alopecia, numbness, photosensitivity,
black tongue

**Special Nursing Considerations
and Patient Education**
- Monitor blood pressure, both lying and standing;
  notify physician if systolic is less than 20 mm Hg.
- Assess weight each week.
- Increase fluids and bulk.
- Administer at hs if sedation occurs.
- Offer sugar-free candy to relieve dry mouth.
- Provide safety measures; assist with ambulation.
- Be certain that patient swallows the medication.
- Monitor output.
- Arrange for blood studies if on long-term
  treatment.
- Teach patient to
  – wear sunscreen.
  – avoid alcohol and OTC medications.
  – not discontinue without physician's order.
  – use caution when driving.
  – that therapeutic effects may take 2–3 weeks.
  – change position slowly.

271

Nystatin

Brand Name
Mycostatin, Nilstat

Actions
Antibiotic, antifungal; causes leakage of essential
components through walls of susceptible
organisms.

Uses
Candida albicans infections

Contraindications
Hypersensitivity

Interactions
None

Dose
Adult   PO: 500,000–1,000,000 U tid
Peds   PO: 100,000–600,000 U qid

Forms
Cream, ointment, powder, suspension, tablets,
vaginal suppositories and tablets

Adverse Effects
Diarrhea, GI distress, nausea, vomiting

**Special Nursing Considerations
and Patient Education**
- Avoid contact with drugs by hands.
- Protect liquid form from heat and light, use within
  1 week.
- Do not mix suspensions in foods.
- Give infants ½ of a dose in each side of mouth, to
  be retained as long as possible.
- Teach patient
    - to continue vaginal tablets when menstruating.
    - to continue treatment at least 48 hours after
      syptoms are gone.
    - to maintain good personal hygiene.
    - to refrain from sexual intercourse during
      treatment.

Oxazepam

Brand Name
Serax

Actions
Antianxiety, hypnotic, sedative, tranquilizer. Onset evident in 1–2 hours.

Uses
Acute alcohol withdrawal, anxiety, insomnia

Contraindications
Meds Alcohol, CNS depressants
Other Acute narrow-angle glaucoma, children, psychosis. *Use with caution:* Allergy to chemically related medications, epilepsy, hepatic or renal impairment, pulmonary disease

Interactions
Antihistamines, barbiturates, cimetidine, MAO inhibitors, narcotics, phenothiazines, tricyclic antidepressants

Dose
Adult 10–30 mg tid–qid

Forms
Capsules, tablets

Adverse Effects
Ataxia, drowsiness, edema, euphoria,
hypotension, lethargy, speech slurring, tremors
**Special Nursing Considerations
and Patient Education**
- Protect medication from direct light.
- Encourage patient to verbalize feelings of anxiety.
- Be aware that
  - medication can be addictive; when
    discontinued, decrease dosage gradually.
- Teach patient to
  - be cautious when driving or involved in
    potentially hazardous tasks.
  - notify physician for ecchymosis, eye pain, fever,
    hemorrhage, sore throat.
  - take with food.
  - change position slowly.

Oxycodone/Acetamnophen

Brand Name
Percocet, Tylox

Actions
Narcotic analgesic—controlled substance II.
Onset evident in 10–15 minutes.

Uses
Moderate—severe pain

Contraindications
Hypersensitivity, addictive individuals. *Use with caution:* head injury, increased intracranial pressure, acute abdominal conditions, elderly or debilitated patients, severe hepatic or renal impairment, hypothyroidism, Addison's disease, prostatic hypertrophy

Interactions
MAO inhibitors, anticholinergics, CNS depressants

Dose
Adult   PO: 2.5–5 mg q6h prn
Peds   PO: over 12 yr: 2.5 mg q6h prn; 6–12 yr: 1.25 mg q6h prn

Forms
Tablets

Adverse Effects
Respiratory depression, urinary retention, lightheadedness, dizziness, sedation, nausea, vomiting, euphoria, dysphoria, constipation, hypotension, physical and psychological dependence

Special Nursing Considerations and Patient Education
- Assess I&O, vital signs.
- Evaluate pain status.
- Provide safety measures.
- Offer emotional support.
- Overdose: Narcan is antidote.
- Withdraw medication slowly.
- Teach patient
  - that dependence may occur.
  - to take only as ordered.
  - to avoid driving.

Oxytocin

Brand Name
Pitocin, Syntocinon

Actions
Hormone; Increases permeability of sodium ions
in uterine cells leading to increased numbers of
contracting myofibrils. Onset evident: buccal 30
minutes; IM 3–7 minutes; IV 1 minute.

Uses
Labor induction, uterine hemorrhage or inertia

Contraindications
Amniotic fluid embolism, cephalopelvic
disproportion, children, fetal distress or
malpresentation, first stage labor, hyper- or
hypotonic uterine contractions, severe medical
conditions or toxemia, thromboplastin
predisposition, uterine overdistention

Interactions
None

Dose
Adult   Individualized; 10–40 U in 1,000 cc of 5%
dextrose

Forms
Citrate buccal tablets; synthetic injection and
nasal spray

Adverse Effects

Fetus   Bradycardia, death, dysrhythmias, hypoxia, internal hemorrhage

Mother   Convulsions, dysrhythmias, hypertensive crisis, hypotension, pelvic hematoma, tetanic uterine contractions, uterine rupture

Special Nursing Considerations
and Patient Education

- Administer only 1 route at a time.
- Do not give IV in undiluted form or in high concentration.
- Administer medication exactly as directed.
- Monitor patient constantly for duration and frequency of contractions, fetal heart rate and tone, I&O, vital signs.
- Report contractions that are excessively long (over 90 seconds) or strong (50 mm Hg).

Papaverine HCl

Brand Name
   Cerebid, Cerespan, Pavabid

Actions
   Antispasmodic, peripheral vasodilator; relaxes
   peripheral blood vessels. Onset evident in 30–60
   minutes.

Uses
   Cerebral, myocardial, or peripheral ischemia;
   circulatory disorders (blood vessel spasm)

Contraindications
Meds   Alcohol
Other   Children, complete A-V block, smoking. *Use
      with caution:* Circulatory dysfunction, coro-
      nary insufficiency, CVA, glaucoma, MI

Dose
Adult   Individualized; PO: 100–300 mg 3–5x/day
      (sustained-release forms) or 150 mg q12h

Forms
   Injection, long-acting capsules, tablets

Adverse Effects
   Anorexia, constipation, diarrhea, dizziness,
   flushing, headache, nausea, sedation, sweating,
   vomiting

**Special Nursing Considerations
and Patient Educations**
- Protect medication from heat and light.
- Do not mix medication with Ringer's Lactate.
- Do not crush long-acting capsules.
- Administer IV dose over 1–2 minutes.
- Administer with meals.
- Monitor blood pressure, pulse, respirations
  (parenteral use).
- Teach patient
  - to be cautious when driving or involved in
    potentially hazardous tasks.
  - to use caution during exercise to avoid
    dizziness.
  - to stop smoking.

Penicillin V Potassium

Brand Name
Pen-Vee K, V-Cillin K

Actions
Antibiotic, anti-infective; hinders ability of bacteria to synthesize cell walls.

Uses
Infections (gonococci, pneumococci, staphylococci, streptococci), rheumatic fever, surgery

Contraindications
Allergy to any penicillin. *Use with caution:* Allergy to cephalosporins, general allergies

Interactions
Chloramphenicol, erythromycin, neomycin, paromomycin, tetracycline, troleandomycin

Dose
Adult   250–500 mg tid–qid
Peds   15–50 mg/kg in 3–6 divided doses

Forms
Capsules, pediatric drops or suspension, solution, suspension, tablets

Adverse Effects
Anemia, black "hairy" tongue, diarrhea, nausea, superinfections, vomiting

Special Nursing Considerations
and Patient Education
- Administer 1 hour before or 2 hours after meals.
- Have out-patient stay for 30 minutes after
  receiving medication in case of allergic reaction.
- Teach patient
  - that medication may cause tongue to darken.
  - to complete full course of therapy.

Pentazocine HCl

Brand Name
Talwin

Actions
Analgesic, sedative. Onset evident: IM, PO, SC
15–30 minutes; IV 2–3 minutes.

Uses
Pain, sedation

Contraindications
Meds Alcohol, CNS depressants
Other Children under 12, head Injury, Increased
intracranial pressure. *Use with caution:*
Gallbladder disorders, hepatic or renal
dysfunction, MI, narcotic dependence,
prostatic hypertrophy, seizures, urethral
stricture

Interactions
Anticholinergics, antidepressants, hypnotics, MAO
inhibitors, meperidine, methadone, morphine,
narcotics, sedatives, skeletal muscle relaxants,
tranquilizers, tricyclic antidepressants

Dose
Adult PO: initial dose, 50 mg q3–4h; may be
increased to 100 mg; *maximum* dose: 600
mg/day; IM/IV/SC: 30 mg q3–4h; *maximum*
dose: 300 mg/day

Forms
Hydrochloride tablets, lactate injection

Adverse Effects
Blurred vision, diaphoresis, dizziness, drowsiness, dry mouth, nausea, vomiting

Special Nursing Considerations
and Patient Education
- Protect medication from direct light.
- Do not combine with soluble barbiturates in same syringe because precipitations will occur.
- Offer hard candy (regular or sugar-free) to relieve dry mouth.
- Monitor response of medication to pain.
- Be aware that
  - dependence is possible; when discontinued, decrease dosage gradually.
  - tolerance can develop.
  - IM and IV are preferred over SC when frequent injections are needed.
- Teach patient
  - to avoid alcohol and other depressants.
  - to be cautious when driving or involved in potentially hazardous tasks.

Pentobarbital Sodium

Brand Name
  Nembutal

Actions
  Barbiturate, hypnotic, sedative. Onset evident in
  15–20 minutes.

Uses
  Insomnia, sedation

Contraindications
Meds Alcohol, CNS depressants
Other Hepatic or renal disease, porphyria,
      uncontrolled pain. *Use with caution:* Anemia
      (parenteral use), asthma, cardiovascular
      disease, diabetes, epilepsy, hyperkinesis,
      hypertension, hyperthyroidism (parenteral
      use), hypoadrenalism, hypotension, narrow-
      angle glaucoma, pulmonary or renal disease

Interactions
  Chloramphenicol, corticosteroids, digitoxin, doxycycline, estradiol, griseofulvin, isoniazid, MAO inhibitors, oral anticoagulants or contraceptives,
  phenylbutazone, phenytoin, valproic acid

Dose
Adult PO: Hypnotic: 100–200 mg hs; sedative: 20–
      30 mg tid–qid; *maximum* dose: 120 mg/day
Peds PO: 6 mg/kg/day in 3 divided doses

Forms
Capsules, elixir, injection, long-acting tablets, suppositories

Adverse Effects
Apnea, bronchospasm, hypotension, laryngospasm, respiratory depression

Special Nursing Considerations and Patient Education
- Protect elixir from direct light.
- Administer hypnotic 15–30 minutes prior to hs.
- Administer IM dose slowly and deeply (no more than 5 cc at one site); observe for adverse effects for 30 minutes.
- Administer IV dose slowly; monitor vital signs q3–5min.
- Be aware that
  - medication is habit-forming; when discontinued, decrease dosage gradually.
- Teach patient
  - that medication may cause photosensitivity.
  - to be cautious when driving or involved in potentially hazardous tasks.

Pentoxiflylline

Brand Name
Trental

Actions
Homorheologic agent. Onset evident in 2–4
weeks.

Uses
Intermittent claudication.

Contraindications
Xanthines, caffeine, theophylline, theobromine.
Use with caution: coronary artery disease,
cerebrovascular disease

Interactions
Antihypertensives, nitrates, oral anticoagulants

Dose
Adult   PO: 400 mg tid with meals

Forms
Tablets

Adverse Effects
Dyspepsia, nausea, vomiting, flatus, dizziness,
headache, arrhythmia, tremors, angina

**Special Nursing Considerations
and Patient Education**
- Monitor blood pressure, especially if the patient is taking antihypertensives.
- Administer with meals.
- Teach patient to
  - swallow tablet whole.
  - avoid smoking.
  - avoid driving.

Perphenazine

Brand Name
  Trilafon

Actions
  Antiemetic, antipsychotic. Onset evident: PO/IM
  2–6 hrs; IV rapid.

Uses
  Acute or chronic schizophrenia; bipolar
  depression; involutional, senile, or toxic
  psychosis; nausea; vomiting

Contraindications
Meds Alcohol
Other Blood disorders, bone-marrow disorders,
  children under 12, hepatic impairment. *Use
  with caution:* Allergy to phenothiazines,
  cardiovascular disorders, epilepsy,
  glaucoma, Parkinson's disease, peptic ulcer,
  prostatic hypertrophy, respiratory disorder,
  urinary retention

Interactions
  Amphetamines, antacids, anticonvulsants,
  antidiarrheals, antihistamines, atopine-like
  medications, CNS depressants, guanethidine,
  hypnotics, levodopa, MAO inhibitors, methyldopa,
  narcotics, reserpine, sedatives, tranquilizers,
  tricyclic antidepressants

Dose
Adult PO: 4–16 mg/day in 2–4 divided doses; IM:
  5–10 mg q6h; IV: 1mg at 1–2 minute
290 intervals.

Peds Over 12 yr: Same as adult

Forms
Concentrate, injection, prolonged-action tablets, suppositories, syrup, tablets

Adverse Effects
Blurred vision, constipation, dermatitis, dizziness, dry mouth, extrapyramidal symptoms, orthostatic hypotension, sedation, syncope

Special Nursing Considerations and Patient Education
- Protect liquid forms from direct light.
- Do not crush prolonged-action tablets.
- Dilute concentrate; avoid using apple or grape juice, coffee, cola, tea.
- Administer IM dose slowly and deeply; have patient remain recumbent for ½ hour; massage injection site.
- Avoid administering IV dose in undiluted form; administer slowly as directed.
- When discontinued, decrease dosage gradually.
- Monitor for fine vermicular tongue movements (may indicate early tardive dyskinesia).
- Offer hard candy (regular or sugar-free) to relieve dry mouth.
- Teach patient
  - that medication may cause photosensitivity.
  - to be cautious when driving or involved in potentially hazardous tasks.
  - urine may become pink-red in color.

Phenelzine Sulfate

Brand Name
Nardil

Actions
MAO inhibitor. Onset evident in 1–2 weeks.

Uses
Endogenous or reactive depression, involutional melancholia

Contraindications
Meds Alcohol, amphetamines, CNS depressants, dopamine, epinephrine, levodopa, methyldopa, norepinephrine, tryptophan, tyramine
Other Arteriosclerosis, atonic colitis, cardiovascular disease, cerebrovascular disease, children under 16, elderly over 60, epilepsy, hepatic impairment, hypernatremia, hypertension, hyperthyroidism, paranoid schizophrenia, pheochromocytoma. *Use with caution:* Convulsive disorders, glaucoma

Interactions
Antihypertensives, barbiturates, general anesthesia, oral hypoglycemic agents, reserpine, tricyclic antidepressants

Dose
Adult 15 mg tid; *maximum* dose: 75 mg/day; *maintenance* dose: 15 mg qd–qod

Forms
Tablets

Adverse Effects
Constipation, dizziness, drowsiness, dry mouth,
GI disturbances, insomnia, orthostatic
hypotension, tremors

**Special Nursing Considerations
and Patient Education**
- Protect medication from light and heat.
- Use caution when administering to a patient with
  suicidal potential; ensure patient swallows dose.
- When discontinued, decrease dosage gradually.
- Monitor blood pressure, I&O, weight; for diabetic
  patients monitor for evidence of hypoglycemia.
- Offer hard candy (regular or sugar-free) to relieve
  dry mouth.
- Give diet that does not contain foods high in
  tryptophan and tyramine (see Appendix F).
- Teach patient to
  - change position slowly to decrease
    hypotension.
  - limit caffeine intake.
  - continue diet restrictions for 2 weeks after
    medication is discontinued.
  - avoid alcohol, OTC medications.

Phenobarbital,
Phenobarbital Sodium

Brand Name
Phenobarbital, Luminal

Actions
Hypnotic, sedative; reduces nerve impulses to cerebral cortex through action on brainstem reticular formation. Onset evident in 1 hour.

Uses
Insomnia, seizures (focal, grand mal, status epilepticus)

Contraindications
Meds Alcohol, CNS depressants
Other Hepatic dysfunction, latent porphyria. *Use with caution:* Anemia; asthma; borderline hypoadrenalism; cardiac, renal, or hepatic impairment; diabetes; epilepsy; hyperkinesis; hypertension or hyperthyroidism (parenteral use)

Interactions
Anticoagulants, chloramphenicol, corticosteroids, digitoxin, doxycycline, estradiol, griseofulvin, isoniazid, MAO inhibitors, oral contraceptives, phenylbutazone, phenytoin, valproic acid

Dose
Adult PO: Sedative: 16–32 mg; hypnotic: 100 mg hs

Peds   PO: Sedative: 6 mg/kg/day in 3 divided
          doses; hypnotic: 3–6 mg/kg hs

Forms
Elixir, prolonged-action capsules, injection, tablets

Adverse Effects
Apnea, bradycardia, confusion, depression,
diarrhea, dizziness, excitement, nausea,
somnolence, vomiting

**Special Nursing Considerations
and Patient Education**
• Protect liquid forms from light.
• Do not crush prolonged-action capsules.
• Administer IM deeply into muscle.
• When IV form used, monitor patient constantly for
  rapid change in condition.
• Use caution when administering to a patient with
  suicidal potential; ensure patient swallows dose.
• Monitor vital signs, serum levels.
• Be aware that
  – medication can be habit-forming; when
    discontinued, decrease dosage gradually.
  – cross tolerance to barbiturates is possible.
• Teach patient
  – that medication may cause photosensitivity.
  – to notify physician of fever, hemorrhage,
    jaundice, rash, sore throat.
  – to be cautious when driving or involved in
    potentially hazardous tasks.
  – to not discontinue medication abruptly.

Phenylpropanolamine Hydrochloride/Guaifensen

Brand Name
Entex LA

Actions
Decongestant, expectorant.

Uses
Symptomatic relief of sinusitis, bronchitis, pharyngitis and corza when associated with nasal congestion

Contraindications
MAO inhibitors, hypersensitivity to sympathomimetics. Severe hypertension. *Use with caution:* hypertension, diabetes mellitus, increased intraocular pressure, hyperthyroidism, prostatic hypertrophy

Interactions
MAO inhibitors

Dose
Adult PO: 1 tablet q12h
Peds   PO: ½ tablet q12h

Forms
Tablets

Adverse Effects
Nervousness, insomnia, restlessness, headache,
gastric irritation

**Special Nursing Considerations
and Patient Education**
• Teach patient to
  – swallow tablet whole; do not crush or chew.

Phenytoin, Phenytoin Sodium

Brand Name
Dilantin, Dilantin Infantab, Dilantin 30 Pediatric

Actions
Anticonvulsant; promotes sodium efflux from
neurons, which then hinders motor cortex seizure
activity. Onset evident: PO 8 hours; IV 5 minutes.

Uses
Digitalis-induced dysrhythmias, grand mal or
psychomotor seizures, migraine or trigeminal
neuralgia pain

Contraindications
Meds Alcohol
Other Adams-Stokes syndrome, atrioventricular
block, hepatic disease, sinoatrial block, sinus
bradycardia

Interactions
Antidepressants, antihistamines, aspirin,
barbiturates, chloramphenicol, chlordiazepoxide,
CNS depressants, corticosteroids, cortisone,
cycloserine, digitalis, disulfiram, doxycycline,
estrogens, folic acid antagonists, glutethemide,
griseofulvin, hypnotics, hypoglycemics, isoniazid,
levodopa, lidocaine, methotrexate, methyl-
phenidate, oral anticoagulants or contraceptives,
oxyphenbutazone, para-aminosalicylic acid,

298

phenothiazines, phenylbutazone, propranolol, quinidine, sedatives, sulfa medications, sympathomimetics, tranquilizers, tubocurarine, valproic acid

Dose
Adult PO: initial dose, 100 mg tid; *maintenance* dose: 300–600 mg/day

Peds PO: initial dose, 5 mg/kg/day in 2–3 divided doses; *maximum* dose: 300 mg/day; *maintenance* dose: 4–8 mg/kg/day

Forms
Capsules, injection, suspension, tablets

Adverse Effects
Ataxia, confusion, constipation, dizziness, extrapyramidal symptoms, gingival hyperplasia, hallucinations, headache, insomnia, nausea, nervousness, nystagmus, tremors, vomiting

Special Nursing Considerations and Patient Education
- Administer exactly as directed; do not exceed 50 mg/minute; follow injection with saline to avoid irritation of vein.
- Take pulse prior to administration of IV dose and compare with patient's guidelines.
- Administer IM dose deep into large muscle.
- Administer oral dose with a ½ glass of water immediately before or after meals to decrease GI distress.

(continued)

Phenytoin, Phenytoin Sodium
(continued)

- Monitor blood pressure, pulse, respiration; for diabetic patients, monitor for signs of hyperglycemia (see Appendix B).
- When discontinued, decrease dosage gradually.
Be aware that
  - there is a small margin between therapeutic and toxic levels.
- Teach patient
  - that medication may turn urine brown, pink, or red.
  - to avoid alcohol.
  - to notify physician if patient becomes ill, and for fever, rash, sore throat.
  - to be cautious when driving or involved in potentially hazardous tasks.
  - to maintain proper oral hygiene because of possible gingival hyperplasia.
- Teach patient and family
  - regarding possibility of seizures.

Notes

_____

_____

_____

_____

_____

_____

_____

_____

_____

_____

_____

_____

_____

_____

_____

_____

_____

_____

Piroxicam

Brand Name
Feldene

Actions
Non-steroidal anti-inflammatory, analgesic, antipyretic. Onset evident: analgesic 4 hours; anti-inflammatory 14 days.

Uses
Acute and chronic rheumatoid arthritis, osteoarthritis, mild to moderate pain.

Contraindications
Hypersensitivity, cardiac disorders, hyperthyroidism, diabetes mellitus, angioedema, GI bleeding, ulcers. *Use with caution:* cardiovascular, hepatic and renal diseases

Interactions
Coumadin, phenytoin, sulfanamides, aspirin, phenobarbital, oral anticoagulants, oral hypoglycemics, probenecid, diuretics, lithium

Dose
Adult   PO: 20 mg qd

Forms
Capsules

Adverse Effects
GI discomfort (e.g., diarrhea, nausea and vomiting, constipation, abdominal pain), edema, dizziness, headache, rash, vertigo, tinnitus, pruritus, anxiety, drowsiness, flatulence, fluid retention, UTI, thirst, eye irritation

Special Nursing Considerations and Patient Educations
- Administer with food and milk.
- Assess pain—location, duration, type—prior to and during therapy.
- Assess for increased joint movement.
- Teach patient to
  - avoid driving.
  - take with water and remain upright for 30 minutes.
  - notify physician if rash, fever, chills, visual problems, or edema occur.

Potassium Chloride

Brand Name
Slow-K, Kaon-Cl, Kato, Kay-Ciel, K-Lor, K-Tab, Klorvess, Micro-K, Klor-Con, Kolyum

Actions
Electrolyte—potassium salt. Onset evident: IV rapid; PO 30 minutes.

Uses
Correction and prevention of potassium deficiency, cardiac arrhythmias due to cardiac glycoside toxicity

Contraindications
Allergy to tortrazine, aspirin, severe renal impairment, hyperkalemic, untreated Addison's disease acute dehydration, digitalized patients. *Use with caution:* cardiac disease

Interactions
Potassium phosphate IV, calcium and magnesium products, potassium sparing diuretics, captopril, enalapril, salt substitutes with potassium salts, anticholinergics

Dose
Adult PO: prevention: 20 mEq/day in divided doses; treatment: 40–100 mEq/day in divided doses; IV: 10–20 mEq/hour; *maximum* dose:150 mEq/day

Peds IV, PO: 2–3 mEq/kg/day or 40 mEq/m²/day

Forms
  IV solution, tablets, powder (also sugar-free)

Adverse Effects
  Hyperkalemia, nausea, vomiting, diarrhea,
  abdominal discomfort, GI obstruction, GI bleeding,
  rash, arrhythmias, weakness, restlessness,
  confusion, paralysis, cramps, ulceration of small
  bowel, oliguria, cold extremities

**Special Nursing Considerations
and Patient Education**
- Administer IV slowly; do not give bolus or IM.
- Monitor serum potassium level during treatment.
- Monitor I&O.
- Notify physician if urine output decreases.
- Monitor vital signs, cardiac status (rate, rhythm).
- Dissolve powder fully in 120 ml of water.
- Agitate IV solution to decrease layering.
- Do not add to hanging IV bottle.
- Teach patient to
  - modify diet with potassium-rich foods.
  - avoid OTC medications—antacids, salt
    substitutes, analgesics, vitamins.
  - swallow, not chew, tablets.
  - report signs and symptoms of hyperkalcemia.
  - wax matrix may be found in stool.
  - take missed dose within 2 hours, or wait until
    next dose; do not take double dose.

Potassium Salts

Brand Name
Potassium bicarbonate: K-lyte, Micro-K Potassium chloride: K-tab, Kaon-cl, Klor-vess, Micro-K, Slow-K, Kay-Ciel, K-lor; Potassium gluconate: Kaopn, Tri-K, Twin-K, Kaylixir

Actions
Electrolyte. Onset: IV rapid; PO 30 minutes.

Uses
Prevention or treatement of potassium depletion, cardiac arrhythmias

Contraindications
Hyperkalemia, renal impairment, Addison's disease, severe tissue trauma, acute dehydration
Use with caution cardiac disorders

Interactions
Products with calcium or magnesium, potassium-sparing diuretics, salt substitutes, captopril, digitalis, anticholinergics

Dose
Adult PO: prevention: 20 mEq/day bid or qid; treatment: 40–100 mEq/day bid or qid; IV: 10–20 mEq/hour; *maximum* dose: 150 mEq/day

Peds PO/IV: 2–3 mEq/kg/day

Forms
Tablets, injection for IV, powder

Adverse Effects
Arrhythmias, nausea and vomiting, diarrhea, abdominal pain, cramps, rash, oliguria, confusion, GI obstruction, GI bleeding, hyperkalemia

Special Nursing Considerations and Patient Education
- Monitor potassium level during treatment.
- Monitor I &O, cardiac status.
- Administer IV slowly (10–20 mEq/hour); do not give IM or IV bolus.
- Administer with meals.
- Agitate IV preparation solution.
- Use only clear solutions.
- Teach patient to
  - notify physician with signs and symptoms of hyperkalemia.
  - dissolve tablet or powder in at least 120 cc of liquid; drink slowly.
  - not chew or crush tablets.
  - not use salt substitutes.
  - disregard wax matrix in stool.
  - not double doses if dose is forgotten.
  - follow prescribed diet.

Prazosin Hydrochloride

Brand Name
Minipress

Actions
Antihypertensive, alpha-adrenergic blocker. Onset
evident in 2 hours.

Uses
Hypertension, Raynaud's vasospasm, CHF

Contraindications
Hypersensitivity

Interactions
Beta-blockers, nitroglycerine, oral anticoagulants.
Use with caution: renal failure

Dose
Adult PO: initial dose: 1 mg bid/tid; *maintenance*
dose: 6–15 mg qd in divided doses

Forms
Capsules

Adverse Effects
Dizziness, headache, drowsiness, lack of energy,
weakness, palpitations, nausea, syncope, depression, orthostatic hypotension, abdominal cramps,
blurred vision, dry mouth

Special Nursing Considerations
and Patient Education

- Have patient lie in recumbent position if syncope occurs.
- Offer emotional support if syncope occurs.
- Monitor vital signs, blood pressure, edema.
- Observe for signs and symptoms of CHF.
- Administer first dose at hs.
- Observe for signs of dizziness, weakness and syncope; provide safety precautions.
- Teach patient to
  - avoid OTC medications.
  - notify physician if side effects occur.
  - lie down if dizziness occurs.
  - change position slowly.
  - follow diet, exercise regimen.
  - avoid driving.

Prednisone

Brand Name
Deltasone, Sterapred

Actions
Anti-inflammatory; inhibits immune response

Uses
Allergies; collagen, dermatologic, respiratory, or rheumatic diseases; hematologic or ophthalmologic disorders; palliative measure for leukemia; primary or secondary adrenocortical insufficiency

Contraindications
Active tuberculosis, eye infections due to herpes simplex virus, infections uncontrolled by antibiotics, psychosis, systemic fungal infection. *Use with caution:* Cardiac disorder, cirrhosis, diabetes, emotional instability, fresh intestinal anastomosis, glaucoma, hepatic dysfunction, herpes simplex (ocular), history of tuberculosis, hypertension, hypothyroidism, myasthenia gravis, osteoporosis, peptic ulcer, pyrogenic infections, renal insufficiency, ulcerative colitis

Interactions
Aspirin, ephedrine, insulin, oral anticoagulants or hypoglycemic agents, phenobarbital, phenytoin, potassium-depleting diuretics, rifampin

310

Dose

Adult Initial dose: 30–60 mg/day in 2–4 divided
doses; after 2–7 days, *decrease gradually* by
5–10 mg to a *maintenance* dose of 5–20 mg/
day

Peds Initial dose: 2 mg/kg/day in 4 divided doses;
decrease gradually over 2–3 weeks to a
maintenance dose of 1.5 mg/kg/day

Forms

Tablets

Adverse Effects

Abdominal distention, blurred vision, electrolyte
disturbance, hypotension, increased intracranial
pressure, mood changes, nausea, osteoporosis,
petechiae, purpura, vomiting

**Special Nursing Considerations
and Patient Education**

- Protect medication from air and direct light.
- Monitor weight, potassium levels periodically.
- Be aware that
  - dependence is possible; when discontinued,
    decrease dosage gradually.
- Teach patient to
  - ingest a diet high in potassium and protein but
    low in salt.
  - take medications after meals and at hs.
  - carry some type of Medic Alert card or bracelet.
  - avoid stress as much as possible.
  - notify physician of abdominal pain, confusion,
    hypotension, illness, possible infections.

311

Procainamide HCl

Brand Name
Pronestyl

Actions
Antidysrhythmic; decreases cardiac automaticity, conductivity, and excitability. Onset evident: PO: 30 minutes; IV immediately.

Uses
Digitalis intoxication, dysrhythmias (atrial fibrillation, paroxysmal atrial tachycardia, premature ventricular contractions, ventricular tachycardia)

Contraindications
Allergies, blood dyscrasias, cardiac damage, complete atrioventricular heart block, myasthenia gravis, 2nd or 3rd degree atrioventricular block. *Use with caution:* Allergy to chemically related medications; asthma; hepatic or renal dysfunction; lupus erythematosus

Interactions
Ammonium chloride, cholinergics, digitalis, isoniazid, lidocaine, skeletal muscle relaxants, sodium bicarbonate

Dose
Adult   PO: initial dose: 1 gm; *maintenance* dose: 50 mg/kg/day q3h
Peds   PO: 50 mg/kg in 4–6 divided doses

312

Forms
Capsules, injection, tablets

Adverse Effects
Anorexia, depression, diarrhea, hallucinations, lupus erythematosis syndrome, nausea, psychosis, urticaria, vomiting

**Special Nursing Considerations
and Patient Education**
- Discard solutions if darker than light amber or otherwise discolored.
- Protect vials from light and temperature changes.
- Discontinue if diastolic blood pressure is below 15 mm Hg.
- Monitor urinary output, vital signs; with IV, constantly monitor blood pressure, EKG.
- Be aware that
  - plasma levels should be 4–8 mcg/ml.
  - that medication is cumulative.
- Teach patient
  - to take with food to decrease GI upset.
  - to decrease intake of caffeine and iced drinks because of their stimulant effect.
  - that medication may cause a bitter taste in mouth.
  - to carry some type of Medic Alert card or bracelet.
  - to be cautious when driving or involved in potentially hazardous tasks.
  - to notify physician of fever, hemorrhage, rash, respiratory tract infection, sore throat.
  - to take around the clock.

313

Prochlorperazine Edisylate/ Prochlorperazine Maleate

Brand Name
Compazine, Chlorazine

Actions
Antiemetic. Onset evident: PO 30–40 minutes; rectal 60 minutes; IM 10–20 minutes.

Uses
Control of severe nausea and vomiting, acute and chronic psychosis, nonpsychotic anxiety

Contraindications
Comatose states, presence of large amounts of CNS depressants, bone marrow suppression, seizures, hypersensitivity to phenothiazines. *Use with caution:* glaucoma, epilepsy, CNS tumors, respiratory diseases, impaired cardiovascular symptoms

Interactions
Antacids, anticholinergics, antidepressants, antiparkinson medications, barbiturates, thiazide diuretics, propranolol

Dose
Adult   PO: 5–10 mg tid/qid or 10 mg tid extended-release; IM: 5–10 mg q3–4h; rectal: 25 mg bid

Peds   PO:Rectal: 18–39 kg: 2.5 mg tid; 14–17 kg:
2.5 mg bid/tid; 9–13 kg: 2.5 mg 1–2 x/day;
IM: 0.13 mg/kg in a single dose

Forms
Oral solution, tablets, injection, extended-release
capsules

Adverse Effects
Drowsiness, dizziness, blurred vision, hypotension, extrapyramidal reactions, agitation, insomnia, dystonias, pseudoparkinsonism, tardive
dyskinesia, contact dermatitis, depression, euphoria, photosensitivity, dry mouth, constipation

Special Nursing Considerations
and Patient Education
- Do not crush or chew extended-release capsules.
- Offer emotional support.
- Assess nausea and vomiting prior to and during
  treatment.
- Monitor mental status.
- Assess vital signs and blood pressure.
- Observe for extrapyramidal symptoms and tardive
  dyskinesia—notify physician if either occur.
- Administer IM slowly in deep muscle; have patient
  lie down for 30 minutes after injection.
- Inform patient that symptoms of tardive
  dyskinesia are temporary and reversible.
- Teach patient to
  - use sunscreen.
  - take as prescribed.
  - use hard, sugar-free candy to relieve dry
    mouth.

315

Promazine HCl

Brand Name
  Sparine

Actions
  Sedative, tranquilizer. Onset evident: PO 1–2
  hours; IM 15 minutes.

Uses
  Alcohol-induced hallucinations, delirium tremens,
  drug withdrawal, nausea, psychosis, vomiting

Contraindications
Meds Alcohol
Other Blood disorders, bone-marrow disorders,
        children under 12. *Use with caution:* Cardiac
        disease, epilepsy, hepatic or respiratory
        disease, parkinsonism, peptic ulcer, prostatic
        hypertrophy

Interactions
  Amphetamines, antacids, anticonvulsants,
  antidiarrheals, antihistamines, atropine-like
  medications, CNS depressants, guanethidine,
  hypnotics, levodopa, MAO Inhibitors, methyldopa,
  narcotics, reserpine, sedatives, tranquilizers,
  tricyclic antidepressants

Dose
Adult PO: 10–200 mg q4–6h; *maximum* dose:
        1,000 mg/day
Peds PO: Over 12 yr: 10–25 mg q4–6h

Forms
Concentrate, injection, syrup, tablets

Adverse Effects
Constipation, drowsiness, extrapyramidal
symptoms, leukopenia, orthostatic hypotension,
sedation, syncope

**Special Nursing Considerations
and Patient Education**
- Protect medication from direct light.
- Administer injections slowly; have patient lie down
  for 30 minutes after administration.
- Dilute concentrate with carbonated drinks or fruit
  juices.
- When discontinued, decrease dosage gradually.
- Monitor for fine vermicular tongue movements
  (may indicate early tardive dyskinesia).
- Teach patient
  - to change position slowly to decrease
    hypotension.
  - that medication may cause photosensitivity.
  - that urine may turn pink or purple.
  - to be cautious when driving or involved in
    potentially hazardous tasks.
  - to use caution in hot weather because of
    potential orthostatic hypotension.

Propoxyphene HCl

Brand Name
Darvon

Actions
Analgesic; increases pain threshold. Onset
evident in 15–30 minutes.

Uses
Pain

Contraindications
Alcohol, children, CNS depressants. *Use with
caution:* Hepatic or renal disease

Interactions
Alcohol, carbamazepine, CNS depressants, oral
anticoagulants, orphenadrine

Dose
Adult   65 mg qid

Forms
Capsules

Adverse Effects
Constipation, dizziness, drowsiness, headache,
nausea, sedation, vomiting

**Special Nursing Considerations
and Patient Education**
- Determine doseage intervals by patient's
  response to pain relief.
- Be aware that
  - dependence is possible; when discontinued,
    decrease dosage gradually.
  - tolerance can develop.
- Teach patient to
  - decrease smoking as it affects drug
    metabolism.
  - be cautious when driving or involved in
    potentially hazardous tasks.

Propranolol

Brand Name
Inderal

Actions
Antianginal, antidysrhythmic, antihypertensive, beta-adrenergic blocking agent. Onset evident: PO 30 minutes–1 hour; IV 3–5 minutes.

Uses
Adjunct for pheochromocytoma, angina pectoris, cardiac dysrhythmias, hypertension, hypertrophic subaortic stenosis, migraine

Contraindications

Meds Adrenergic-augmenting psychotropics, alcohol, furazolidone, general anesthetics, MAO inhibitors

Other Atrioventricular heart block, bronchial asthma, children, congestive heart failure, hypotension, rhinitis, right ventricular failure, sinus bradycardia. *Use with caution:* Bradycardia, bronchospasm (nonallergic), cardiovascular disease, diabetes, emphysema, hay fever, hepatic or renal impairment, hyperthyroid, hypoglycemia, Reynaud's syndrome, Wolff-Parkinson-White syndrome

Interactions
Aminophylline, anti-inflammatories, cimetidine, digitalis, dobutamine, dopamine, guanethidine, isoproterenol, MAO inhibitors, norepinephrine, oral antidiabetics, phenytoin, reserpine

320

Dose
Adult   PO: Initial dose: 10–20 mg tid–qid;
          maintenance dose: 160–640 mg/day

Forms
  Injection, tablets

Adverse Effects
  Bradycardia, congestive heart failure,
  constipation, depression, diarrhea, hallucinations,
  hypoglycemia, lethargy, nausea, orthostatic
  hypotension, respiratory distress, vomiting

**Special Nursing Considerations
and Patient Education**
• Protect medication from light.
• Take apical/radial pulse prior to administration and
  compare with patient's guidelines.
• Administer IV dose slowly.
• Give oral medication before meals and at hs.
• Monitor blood pressure, I&O, neurologic status,
  renal function, vital signs, weight.
• For IV route, withhold other medications for 4
  hours after dose; monitor EKG.
• Have atropine available in case of hypotension.
• When discontinued, decrease dosage gradually.
• Teach patient to
  – decrease caffeine and smoking because of their
    impact on blood pressure.
  – be cautious when driving or involved in
    potentially hazardous tasks.
  – be cautious in cold weather and during
    strenuous exercise because of their impact on
    circulation.
  – notify physician for edema, respiratory distress,
    or illness.
  – change position slowly.   321

Pseudoephedrine HCl/Triprolidine HCl

Brand Name
Actifed

Actions
Antihistamine, decongestant

Uses
Allergic or vasomotor rhinitis, upper respiratory difficulties

Contraindications
Hypersensitivity. *Use with caution:* Hypertension

Interactions
Ephedrine, stimulants

Dose
Adult   10 cc or 1 tablet tid–qid
Peds   1.25–5 cc tid–qid

Forms
Syrup, tablets

Adverse Effects
Drowsiness, stimulation

**Special Nursing Considerations
and Patient Education**
- Protect medication from direct light.
- Teach patient
  - to be cautious when driving or involved in
    potentially hazardous tasks.

Quinidine

Brand Name
Cin-Quin, Quinora

Actions
Antidysrhythmic; delays electrical impulse transmission; decreases pacemaker activity. Onset evident In 1–3 hours.

Uses
Atrial flutter, nocturnal cramps, paroxysmal atrial fibrillation, paroxysmal atrial or ventricular tachycardia, premature atrial or ventricular contractions

Contraindications
Atrioventricular block, digitalis intoxication, dysrhythmia, history of thrombocytopenic purpura, intraventricular conduction defects. *Use with caution:* Acute infections, asthma, bradycardia, cardiac enlargement, chronic valvular disease, congestive heart failure, coronary occlusion, hepatic or renal insufficiency, history of angina pectoris or hyperthyroidism, hypokalemia, incomplete AV block, MI, myasthenia gravis, psoriasis, subacute endocarditis

Interactions
Acetazolamide, antacids, anticholinergics, digoxin, neuromuscular-blocking agents, oral anticoagulants, phenobarbital, phenytoin, rifampin, sodium bicarbonate, thiazide diuretics, verapamil, warfarin

324

Dose

Adult Individualized; PO: 1-2 sustained-release tablets q8–12h; IM: initial dose, 600 mg, then 400 mg q2h

Peds PO: Test dose of 2 mg/kg; *therapeutic* dose: 6 mg/kg/5x/day

Forms

Gluconate or sulfate injection, sulfate tablets, sustained-release tablets containing gluconate or sulfate

Adverse Effects

Bradycardia, cinchonism, confusion, hypotension, nausea, syncope, vomiting

Special Nursing Considerations and Patient Education

- Protect medication from heat and light.
- Take blood pressure, apical pulse rate and rhythm, radial pulse (one minute) prior to administration and compare with patient's guidelines.
- Monitor I&O, serum concentration of medication.
- Administer 1 hour before or 2 hours after meals to maximize absorption.
- Give with food (but not with a full meal) to decrease GI upset.
-

Be aware that
- sustained-release tablets should be taken only for maintenance and prophylaxis.
• Teach patient
- to decrease caffeine intake and smoking because of their stimulant effect.
- to carry a Medic Alert card or bracelet.
- to change position slowly to decrease hypotension.
- may cause a bitter taste in mouth.
- to notify physician of fever, hemorrhage, rash, tinnitus, visual disturbances.
- medication may cause photosensivity.

Notes

Ranitidine

Brand Name
Zantac

Action
Antihistamine; inhibits gastric acid secretion

Uses
Short-term treatment of active duodenal ulcers,
benign gastric ulcers, and gastroesophageal
reflux disease; Zollenger-Ellison Syndrome

Contraindications
Hypersensitivity

Interactions
Antacids, smoking

Dose
Adult   Short-term treatment: PO: 100–150 mg bid
or 300 mg hsx 4–8 weeks; IM/IV: 50 mg q6–
8h; *maximum* dose: 400 mg/day; active ulcer
or hypersecretory conditions: PO: 150 mg
bid; *maximum* dose: 6g/day

Forms
Tablets, injection, IV

Adverse Effects
Headache, malaise, dizziness, bradycardia, rash,
nausea and vomiting

**Special Nursing Considerations
and Patient Education**
- Administer with meals.
- Administer antacids 1 hour before or after meals.
- Evaluate mental status.
- Evaluate GI status.
- Administer IV infusion over at least 5 minutes.
- Administer IM deep into large muscle group.
- False-positive tests for urine protein may occur.
- Teach patient
  - to not take non-prescription medications without notifying physician.
  - to notify physician if side effects occur.
  - that impotence and breast enlargement may occur, but are reversible when therapy is discontinued.

Reserpine

Brand Name
Serpasil

Actions
Antihypertensive, tranquilizer; lessens
catecholamine depletion from peripheral tissues

Uses
Hypertension, psychiatric conditions

Contraindications
Meds   Alcohol, CNS depressants
Other   Active peptic ulcer, depression, ECT,
ulcerative colitis. *Use with caution:*
Gallstones; GI disorders; history of
depression or peptic ulcer; renal insufficiency

Interactions
Anticonvulsants, antihistamines, digitalis,
hypnotics, MAO Inhibitors, narcotics, oral
anticoagulants, phenothiazines, propranolol,
quinidine, sedatives, tranquilizers

Dose
Adult   PO: Initial dose: 0.5 mg/day x 1–2 weeks;
maintenance dose: 0.1–0.25 mg/day
Peds   PO: 0.07 mg/kg/day in 2 divided doses

330

Forms
Capsules, injection, tablets

Adverse Effects
Bradycardia, depression, diarrhea, drowsiness, lethargy, nasal congestion, nausea, weight gain

Special Nursing Considerations and Patient Education
- Protect medication from direct light.
- Check blood pressure prior to administration.
- Administer after meals, or with food/milk, to decrease GI upset.
- Monitor blood pressure, I&O, neurologic status, weight.
- Teach patient to
  - be cautious when driving or involved in potentially hazardous tasks.
  - follow suggested diet.
  - notify physician at first evidence of depression (e.g., early morning insomnia, feeling down, sad affect), or mood changes.
  - avoid alcohol, OTC medications, caffeine.
  - follow hypertension regime: weight reduction, diet, stress management.

Secobarbital Sodium

Brand Name
Seconal

Actions
Hypnotic, sedative; lessens available
norepinephrine. Onset evident: PO 30 minutes;
IM 10–15 minutes.

Uses
Acute convulsive disorders, insomnia, preoperative

Contraindications
Alcohol. *Use with caution:* Anemia, cardiac
disease, diabetes, epilepsy, hyperkinesis,
hypertension, hyperthyroid, hypoadrenalism, pain,
renal or respiratory disease

Interactions
Anticonvulsants; antidepressants; antihistamines;
cortisone, digitalis; digitoxin, griseofulvin;
hypnotics; isoniazid, MAO Inhibitors; narcotics;
oral anticoagulants, contraceptives, or
antidiabetics; phenylbutazone; phenytoin;
sedatives; tranquilizers

Dose
Adult Hypnotic: 100–200 mg PO, IM; sedative:
30–50 mg tid PO
Peds Hypnotic: 3–5 mg/kg PO; sedative: 6 mg/kg/
day PO in 3 divided doses

332

Forms
Capsules, elixir, injection, suppositories, tablets

Adverse Effects
Bradycardia, dizziness, drowsiness, excitement, hypoventilation, nausea, vomiting

Special Nursing Considerations
and Patient Education
- Protect elixir from light.
- Store suppositories in refrigerator.
- Administer IM into deep muscle mass.
- Monitor blood pressure, pulse, respirations: IM for 20–30 minutes; IV constantly, with respirations every 3–5 minutes.
- Be aware that
  - parenteral solutions must be clear.
  - dependence is possible; when discontinued, decrease dosage gradually.
- Teach patient
  - that medication may cause photosensitivity.
  - to be cautious when driving or involved in potentially hazardous tasks.
  - to avoid alcohol, CNS depressants.

Siecralfate

Brand Name
Corafate

Actions
Antiulcer, antipeptic agent. Onset evident in 30 minutes.

Uses
Duodenal ulcer

Contraindications
Hypersensitivity

Interactions
Tetracyclines, cimetidine, phenytoin, digoxin, warfarin, antacids

Dose
Adult: PO: 1 g qid an empty stomach; continue 4–8 weeks

Forms
Tablets

Adverse Effects
Constipation, diarrhea, nausea, gastric discomfort, indigestion, dry mouth, rash, pruritus, back pain, dizziness, vertigo, sleeplessness

Special Nursing Considerations and Patient Education

- Administer medication 1 hour before or 2 hours after meals.
- Assess pain.
- Administer antacids 1/2 hour before or after meals.
- Assess for constipation.
- Provide small, frequent meals.
- Teach patient to
  - take medication as directed.
  - use hard, sugar-free candy to decrease dry mouth.
  - take medication even after feeling better.
  - increase fluids, fiber, bulk to decrease constipation.
  - follow dietary restriction for ulcers.

Spironolactone

Brand Name
Aldactone

Actions
Antihypertensive, potassium-sparing diuretic; blocks selected effects of aldosterone. Onset evident in 1–2 days.

Uses
Edema, adrenal hyperplasia or adenomas, essential hypertension, hypokalimia

Contraindications
Meds Potassium supplements
Other Anuria, hyperkalemia, renal disorders. *Use with caution:* Hepatic disease, renal impairment

Interactions
Anticoagulants, antihypertensives, digitalis glycosides, diuretics, ganglionic blocking agents, norepinephrine, triamterene

Dose
Adult 25–200 mg/day in divided doses
Peds 1.5–3.3 mg/kg/day in 4 divided doses

Forms
  Tablets

Adverse Effects
  Anorexia, ataxia, confusion, cramping, drowsiness
  headache, hyperkalemia, hyponatremia,
  impotence, lethargy, menstrual irregularity,
  nausea

**Special Nursing Considerations
and Patient Education**
- Protect medication from direct light.
- Monitor blood pressure, electrolytes, I&O, weight.
- Observe patient for signs and symptoms of
  hyperkalemia or hyponatremia (see Appendix B).
- Discontinue for electrolyte imbalance.
- Teach patient
    - to avoid potassium-rich foods and salt
      substitutes (see Appendix F).
    - to be cautious when driving or involved in
      potentially hazardous tasks.
    - that full effect of medication does not occur for
      several days.
    - notify physician of gynecomastia, hirsutism,
      hyperkalemia, hyponatremia, impotence,
      menstrual irregularity.
    - to avoid OTC drugs.

Sulindac

Brand Name
Clinoril

Actions
Non-steroidal anti-inflammatory. Onset evident in 7–14 days.

Uses
Rheumatoid arthritis, osteoarthritis, ankylosing spondylitis, acute painful shoulder, acute gouty arthitis

Contraindications
Hypersensitivity, asthma, GI bleeding, ulcers. *Use with caution;* severe cardiovascular, hepatic, ulcer or renal disease

Interactions
Aspirin, oral anticoagulants, oral hypoglycemics, non-steroidal anti-inflammatory agents, probenecid, diuretics, beta-adrenergic blocking agents, lithium, sulfonamides

Dose
Adult   PO: 150–200 mg bid; *maximum* dose: 400 mg/day

Forms
 Tablets

Adverse Effects
 GI pain, dyspepsia, nausea, diarrhea,
 constipation, flatulence, anorexia, rash, dizziness,
 headache, nervousness, edema, tinnitus, cramps,
 fatigue, fluid retention

**Special Nursing Considerations
and Patient Education**
- May administer with food to decrease GI
 discomfort.
- If possible, administer on empty stomach.
- Assess pain—type and location.
- May crush tablets.
- Teach patient to
  - report blurred vision, hearing problems.
  - avoid driving.
  - report changes in output, swelling, pain.
  - not use alcohol, OTC medications or aspirin.
  - remain in upright position 15–30 minutes after
    taking.

Tamoxifen Citrate

Brand Name
Nolvadex

Actions
Antineoplastic; inhibits cell division. Onset evident in 4–10 weeks.

Uses
Treatment of metastatic breast cancer in post-menopausal women, delaying recurrence following total mastectomy and axillary dissection in post-menopausal women.

Contraindications
Hypersensitivity. *Use with caution:* leukopenia, thrombocytopenia

Interactions
None

Dose
Adult: PO: 10–20 mg bid

Forms
Tablets

340

Adverse Effects
   Hot flashes, nausea, vomiting, vaginal bleeding
and discharge, rash, menstrual irregularities, bone
pain, disease flare-up, headache, altered taste,
hypercalcemia

Special Nursing Considerations
and Patient Education
- Inform patient that therapeutic effects take up to
  10 weeks.
- Monitor blood studies and calcium levels prior to
  and during treatment.
- Administer with food to decrease GI discomfort.
- Monitor weight.
- Increase fluid intake.
- Administer analgesics if increased bone pain
  occurs.
- Provide supportive care.
- Teach patient to
  - notify physician of bone pain, lesion flare-ups,
    bleeding.
  - check weight every week.
  - notify physician of suspected pregnancy.
  - use a non-hormonal birth control method.

Temazepam

Brand Name
Restoril, Razepam

Actions
Sedative-hypnotic; benzodiazepine. Onset evident in 30–45 minutes.

Uses
Insomnia (short-term)

Contraindications
Hypersensitivity to benzodiazepines. *Use with caution:* Severe depression, elderly patients, suicidal tendencies, impaired renal or hepatic function, chronic pulmonary insufficiency, narrow-angle glaucoma

Interactions
Cimetidine, disulfiram, alcohol, CNS depressants, antacids

Dose
Adult   PO: 15–30 mg hs

Forms
Capsules

Adverse Effects
Drowsiness, dizziness, lethargy, daytime sedation, confusion, euphoria

342

**Special Nursing Considerations
and Patient Education**

- Monitor amount of medication given to patient to avoid overdose.
- Do not administer within 1 hour of antacids.
- Reduce medication slowly.
- Assess sleeping patterns.
- May administer with food.
- Teach patient to
  - avoid alcohol, OTC medications.
  - avoid driving.
  - not increase dosage without physician's approval.
  - notify physician of suspected pregnancy.
  - take at bedtime.

Terconazole

Brand Name
Terazol 7

Actions
Antifungal, local anti-infective

Uses
Local treatment of vulvovaginal candidiasis

Contraindications
Hypersensitivity

Interactions
None

Dose
Adult   5 g (1 applicator full) intravaginally hs × 7
days

Forms
Cream

Adverse Effects
Headache, vulvovaginal burning, body pain

344

Special Nursing Considerations and Patient Education

- Clean applicator with soap and water after use.
- Teach patient to
  - clean applicator.
  - avoid getting cream in eyes.
  - avoid OTC creams.
  - use full prescribed dose.

Terfendine

Brand Name
  Seldane

Actions
  Antihistamine, anticholinergic, antipruritic. Onset evident in 1–2 hours.

Uses
  Allergy symptoms, rhinitis

Contraindications
  Hypersensitivity. *Use with caution:* prostatic hypertrophy, narrow-angle glaucoma

Interactions
  Antianxiety medications, narcotics, alcohol, sedatives, hypnotics, antidepressants, atropine, haloperidol, phenothiazines

Dose
Adult   PO: 60 mg bid
Peds   PO: under 12 yr: 15 –30 mg bid

Forms
  Tablets

Adverse Effects
  Abdominal pain, bronchospasms, confusion, dry mouth, drowsiness, headache, nausea, nervousness, vomiting, musculoskeletal pain

346

**Special Nursing Considerations
and Patient Education**
- Administer with food to decrease GI problems.
- Provide hard, sugar-free candy to decrease dry mouth.
- Store in light-resistant containers.
- Monitor I&O; observe for urinary retention.
- Teach the patient to
  - be aware of drowsiness; sedation may occur.
  - avoid alcohol.
  - utilize good oral hygiene.
  - utilize humidifier to relieve bronchial secretions.

Tetracycline

Brand Name
Achromycin, Sumycin

Actions
Antiamoebic, antibacterial, antibiotic, antirickettsial; hinders protein synthesis in susceptible microorganisms. Onset evident: PO 1–2 hours; IM/IV rapid.

Uses
Granuloma inguinale, infections caused by gram negative and gram positive bacteria, lymphogranuloma, mycoplasma, ornithosis, psittacosis, rickettsial disease

Contraindications
Meds Antacids, antidiarrheals, dairy products, iron supplements, laxatives containing magnesium
Other History of hepatic disease; renal insufficiency. *Use with caution:* Hepatic or renal disease, lupus erythematosus

Interactions
Cephalosporins, methoxyflurane, oral anticoagulants, penicillins, sodium bicarbonate

Dose
Adult PO: 250 mg q6h; IM: 250–300 mg/day
Peds PO: 25–50 mg/kg/day; IM: 15–25 mg/kg/day

348

Forms
Capsules, injection, ointment, ophthalmic
ointment, pediatric drops, suspension, syrup,
tablets

Adverse Effects
Anorexia, diarrhea, dizziness, nausea, teeth
discoloration (in patients under 8 years), vomiting

**Special Nursing Considerations
and Patient Education**
- Protect medication from light.
- Check expiration date prior to administration.
- Administer oral forms before meals or 2 hours
  after meals with a full glass of water.
- Administer IM dose deep into large muscle mass;
  give IV dose slowly.
- Monitor I&O, weight.
- Continue treatment 24–48 hours after
  temperature is normal.
- Be aware that
  – treatment for beta-hemolytic streptococci-group
    A infections continues for 10 days.
- Teach patient
  – that medication may cause photosensitivity.
  – to be cautious when driving or involved in
    potentially hazardous tasks.
  – to report signs of superinfection: black furry
    tongue, vaginal itching.

Theophylline

Brand Name
Tedral, Elixophyllin, Slo-Phyllin

Actions
Bronchodilator. Onset evident in 15–30 minutes.

Uses
Acute bronchial asthma

Contraindications
Peptic ulcer. *Use with caution:* Acute cardiac disease, cor pulmonale, glaucoma, gout, hepatic or renal disease, hypertension, hyperthyroidism, hypoxemia, myocardial damage, neonates, porphyria, prostatic hypertrophy

Interactions
Acetazolamide, allopurinol, anticoagulants, chlordiazepoxide, cimetidine, clindamycin, digitalis, erythromycin, furosemide, lincomycin, lithium, phenobarbital, phenytoin, propranolol, sympathomimetics

Dose
Adult   PO: 100–200 mg q6h
Peds   PO: 50–100 mg q6h

Forms

Capsules, injection, elixir, suppositories

Adverse Effects

Anorexia, dizziness, headache, insomnia, nausea, palpitations, restlessness, tachycardia, vomiting

**Special Nursing Considerations
and Patient Education**

- Administer medication 1 hour before or 2 hours after meals with a glass of water to decrease GI symptoms.
- Wait 4–6 hours when changing from IV to PO route.
- Monitor I&O, plasma levels, tolerance, vital signs.
- Be aware that
  - serum levels should be within 10–20 μ/cc.
- Teach patient to
  - decrease caffeine intake because it potentiates medication.
  - be cautious when driving or involved in potentially hazardous tasks.
  - not take nonprescription medications without contacting physician.
  - take only as prescribed.

Thioridazine HCl

Brand Name
Mellaril

Actions
Antipsychotic, sedative; hinders dopamine action.
Onset evident in 1 week.

Uses
Behavior problems in children, dementia,
psychosis

Contraindications
Meds Alcohol
Other Cardiac disease. *Use with caution:* Bone-
marrow depression, epilepsy, glaucoma,
hepatic impairment, parkinsonism, prostatic
hypertrophy, respiratory disorders, Reye's
syndrome, urinary retention

Interactions
Amphetamines, antidiarrheals, atropine-like
medications, barbiturates, CNS depressants,
guanethidine, narcotics, phenytoin, tricyclic
antidepressants

Dose
Adult Initial dose, 25–100 mg tid; *maximum* dose:
800 mg/day; *maintenance* dose: 20–200 mg/
day
Peds Over 2 yr: 0.5–3 mg/kg/day

352

Forms
Concentrate, tablets

Adverse Effects
Blurred vision, hypotension, impotence, nausea, sedation, vomiting

**Special Nursing Considerations
and Patient Education**
- Protect liquid form of medication from light.
- Dilute concentrate form per manufacturer's instructions.
- Monitor patient to ensure medication is swallowed.
- When discontinued, decrease dosage gradually.
- Teach patient
  - to be cautious when driving or involved in potentially hazardous tasks.
  - to use caution in hot weather and during strenuous exercise because of potential orthostatic hypotension.
  - to change position slowly to decrease hypotension.
  - that urine may turn pink-red in color.
  - to notify physician of extrapyramidal symptoms or tardive dyskinesia.

Thiothixene HCl

Brand Name
Navane

Actions
Antipsychotic, tranquilizer; depression of brainstem. Onset evident: PO 3 weeks; IM 15–30 minutes.

Uses
Acute or chronic schizophrenia

Contraindications
Meds Alcohol, CNS depressants
Other Blood disorders, children under 12, parkinsonism. *Use with caution:* Cardiovascular disease, epilepsy, glaucoma, hepatic or renal disease, hypertension, peptic ulcer, prostatic hypertrophy, respiratory disorders, Reye's syndrome

Interactions
Amphetamines, antidiarrheals, atropine-like medications, barbiturates, CNS depressants, guanethidine, narcotics, phenytoin, tricyclic antidepressants

Dose
Adult PO: 2–5 mg bid–tid; parenteral: 4 mg bid–qid; *maximum* dose: 60 mg/day

Forms
Capsules, concentrate, injection

Adverse Effects
Blurred vision, constipation, dizziness, drowsiness, dry mouth, extrapyramidal symptoms, hypotension, insomnia

**Special Nursing Considerations
and Patient Education**
• Protect medication from direct light.
• Dilute concentrate form per manufacturer's instructions.
• Avoid contacting medication with hands because of possibility of contact dermatitis.
• When discontinued, decrease dosage gradually.
• Administer IM slowly into deep muscles; have patient remain recumbent for 1/2 hour after administration because of potential orthostatic hypotension.
• Monitor for fine vermicular tongue movements (may indicate early tardive dyskinesia).
• Offer hard candy (regular or sugar-free) to relieve dry mouth.
• Ensure patient swallows medication.
• Monitor BP.
• Teach patient
  – to change position slowly to decrease hypotension.
  – that medication may cause photosensitivity.
  – to be cautious when driving or involved in potentially hazardous tasks.
  – notify physician for hemorrhage, jaundice, rash, sore throat, tremors, vision impairment, weakness.

Thyroid

Brand Name
Armour Thyroid, Thyrolar

Actions
Hormone preparation, increase the metabolic rate of body tissues. Onset: unknown.

Uses
Replacement therapy in hypothyroidism, pituitary TSH suppressants—treatment and prevention of euthyroid goiters, management of thyroid cancer, thyrotoxicosis

Contraindications
Alleriges to active constituents of medicaiton, uncorrected adrenal cortical insufficiency, untreated thyrotoxicosis

Interactions
Oral anticoagulants, insulin, oral hypoglycemics, cholestyramine, estrogen, tricyclic antidepressants

Dose
Adult: PO: myxedema: initial dose: 16 mg/ day × 2 weeks; increase to 32 mg/day × 2–3 weeks; then, 65 mg/day; *maintenance* dose: 65–195 mg/day; hypothyroidism: initial dose: 65 mg/ day; increase by 65 mg q30 days until desired effect achieved

356

Forms
Tablets in 5 potencies

Adverse Effects
Symptoms of hyperthyroidism (e.g., increase pulse pressure, palpitations, tachycardia, headache, tremors, weight loss, menstrual irregularities)

Special Nursing Considerations and Patient Education
- Administer as single dose prior to breakfast.
- Assess cardiac response and status during treatment.
- Schedule regular thyroid function tests.
- Offer emotional support regarding taking the medication for life.
- Teach patient to
  - not stop medication without physician's order.
  - wear medical identification band.
  - avoid OTC medications.
  - keep appointments for regular tests.

Timolol Maleate

Brand Name
Timoptic, Blocadrea

Actions
Beta-adrenergic blocking agent, antihypertensive.
Onset evident: PO unknown; opthalmic 15–30
minutes.

Uses
Hypertension, prevention of MI, chronic stable
angina pectoris, glaucoma, ocular hypertension,
aphakic glaucoma

Contraindications
Hypersentivity, CHF, pulmonary edema,
bradycardia, heart block, asthma, congenital
glaucoma. *Use with caution:* thyrotoxicosis,
hypoglycemia, hepatic impairment

Interactions
Propranolol, metoprolol, nitrates, halothane,
cimitidine, chlorpromazine, oral contraceptives,
thyroid hormones, dopamine, insulin

Dose
Adult　PO: hypertension: 10–20 mg bid; MI: 10mg
bid; opthalmic: instill 1 gtt 0.25–0.5% q d/bid

358

Forms
  Tablets, opthalmic solution

Adverse Effects
  Fatigue, weakness, depression, insomnia,
  diarrhea, nausea and vomiting, bradycardia,
  confusion, anorexia, dyspepsia, rash, dizziness,
  bronchospasm, nasal stuffiness, occular irritation,
  decreased corneal sensitivity, diplopia, ptosis

**Special Nursing Considerations
and Patient Education**
* Assist with comfort measures with eye disease.
* Monitor intraocular pressure periodically.
* Monitor I&O.
* Assess for signs and symptoms of cardiac
  problems.
* Assist with concurrent hypertension therapies
  (diet, exercise, decrease stress).
* Teach patient to
  – consult with physician before stopping
    medication.
  – administer drops appropriately.
  – take medication as directed to avoid withdrawal
    effects.
  – notify physican if side effects occur.

Tolbutamide

Brand Name
Orinase

Actions
Hypoglycemic. Onset evident In 3–6 hours.

Uses
Diabetes, diagnostic test for pancreatic islet cell tumors

Contraindications
Meds Alcohol
Other Acidosis; burns; complicated, diet-controlled, or juvenile diabetes; hepatic or renal insufficiency; ketoacidosis; ketosis. *Use with caution:* Nausea, peptic ulcer, porphyria, thyroid dysfunction, vomiting

Interactions
Anabolic steroids, anti-inflammatories, barbiturates, chloramphenicol, chlorpromazine, corticosteroids, cortisone, coumarin anti-coagulants, pinephrine, estrogens, ethacrynic acid, furosemide, hypnotics, isoniazid, MAO inhibitors, nicotinic acid, oral contraceptives, phenylbutazone, probenecid, propanolol, pyrazinamide, salicylates, sedatives, sulfin-pyrazone, sulfisoxazole, sulfonamides, thiazide diuretics, thyroid preparations

360

Dose
Adult   1–2 gm/day; *maintenance* dose: 0.25–2 gm/
day

Forms
Tablets

Adverse Effects
Anorexia, constipation, diarrhea, dizziness,
headache, hepatic toxicity, hypoglycemia, nausea,
pruritus, vomiting

**Special Nursing Considerations
and Patient Education**
• Monitor for hypoglycemia, urine tests (acetone
and sugar), weight.
• Teach patient
  – that medication may cause breath to be sweet-
smelling.
  – that medication may cause photosensitivity.
  – to check urine daily for sugar and acetone.
  – to follow prescribed diet.
  – to carry some type of Medic Alert card or
bracelet.
  – to not take any new medications without
contacting physician first.
  – to be cautious when driving or involved in
potentially hazardous tasks.
  – to notify physician of indications of
hypoglycemia (e.g., drowsiness, fatigue,
headache).
  – to carry source of glucose (e.g., candy).
  – notify physician for ecchymosis, fever, jaundice,
rash, sore throat.

Trazodone HCl

Brand Name
Desyrel

Actions
Antidepressant. Onset evident in 1–4 weeks.

Uses
Depression

Contraindications
Meds   Anesthetics
Other   Children, ECT, MI (initial recovery phase).
Use with caution: Cardiovascular disease,
suicidal tendencies

Interactions
Alcohol, antihypertensives, barbiturates, CNS
depressants, MAO inhibitors

Dose
Adult   *Initial* dose: 150 mg/day; may be increased
by 50 mg/day q3–4d; *maximum* dose:
inpatient 600 mg/day, outpatient 400 mg/day

Forms
Tablets

Adverse Effects

Blurred vision, confusion, constipation, dizziness
drowsiness, dry mouth, fatigue, hallucinations,
headache, hypotension, incoordination, insomnia,
nausea, nervousness, vomiting

Special Nursing Considerations
and Patient Education

- Administer with or shortly after meals to decrease
  GI irritation.
- Use caution when administering to a patient with
  suicidal potential; ensure patient swallows dose.
- Offer hard candy (regular or sugar-free) to relieve
  dry mouth.
- Teach patient
  - to be cautious when driving or involved in
    potentially hazardous tasks.
  - to take only as prescribed.
  - to notify physician of fainting, light-headedness,
    dizziness.

Tretinoin

Brand name
Retin-A

Actions
Metabolite of vitamin A. Decreases cohesiveness of follicular epithelial cells. Onset evident in 2–6 weeks.

Uses
Acne vulgaris, skin carcinoma

Contraindications
Hypersensitivity

Interactions
Medications: Medications with sulfur, benzoyl peroxide, resorcinol, salicylic acid. *Use with caution:* products with high alcohol concentrations, soaps with drying effects

Dose
Adult   Apply qhs to affected area

Forms
Gel, cream, liquid

Adverse Effects
Skin—redness, edema, blistering, crusted, rash

**Special Nursing Considerations
and Patient Education**
- Apply only to affected area.
- Wash hands after application.
- Avoid applying to mouth, angles of nose, eyes and mucous membranes.
- Teach patient to
  - apply properly.
  - avoid sunlight; use sunscreen.
  - be aware of warmth, peeling and drying.
  - not use shaving lotions or astringents.
  - remove make-up before applying.
  - avoid OTC acne medications while on this treatment.

Triamterene

Brand Name
Dyazide, Dyrenium

Actions
Antihypertensive, potassium-sparing diuretic;
hinders reabsorption of sodium in distal tubule.
Onset evident in 2–4 hours.

Uses
Edema caused by cirrhosis, congestive heart
failure, or hyperaldosteronism; idiopathic or
steroid-induced edema

Contraindications
Meds Lithium, spironolactone
Other Anuria, hepatic disease, hyperkalemia, renal
disorders. *Use with caution:* Diabetes, gout

Interactions
Antihypertensives, digitalis, diuretics,
methotrexate, oral antidiabetics

Dose
Adult Individualized; 100 mg bid; *maximum* dose:
300 mg/day
Peds Individualized; 2–4 mg/kg/day in divided
doses

366

Forms
Capsules

Adverse Effects
Diarrhea, dizziness, electrolyte imbalance,
headache, hyperkalemia, hyponatremia, nausea,
vomiting, weakness

**Special Nursing Considerations
and Patient Education**
- Protect medication from direct light.
- Monitor BP during dosage adjustment; monitor
  I&O, weight.
- Administer medication after meals to decrease GI
  distress.
- When discontinued, decrease dosage gradually to
  prevent rebound kaliuresis.
- Teach patient
  - to avoid potassium-rich foods and salt
    substitutes (see Appendix F).
  - that medication may cause photosensitivity, and
    may color urine blue.
  - to be cautious when driving or involved in
    potentially hazardous tasks.
  - to notify physician for signs and symptoms of
    hyperkalemia, hyponatremia (see Appendix B).

Triazolam

Brand Name
Halcion

Actions
Sedative-hypnotic. Onset evident in 15–30 minutes.

Uses
Short-term management of insomnia, frequent nocturnal or early morning awakening

Contraindications
Hypersensitivity to medication or to other benzodiazepines. *Use with caution:* elderly or debilitated patients, pre-existing CNS depression, suicidal patients, seizure disorders, anemia, renal disease, heptic disease

Interactions
Alcohol, anticonvulsants, antidepressants, antihistamines, levodopa, antacids

Dose
Adult   PO: 0.25–0.5 mg hs; *elderly patients:* 0.125–0.25 mg hs

Forms
Tablets

Adverse Effects
Dizziness, daytime drowsiness, confusion,
headache, paradoxical excitation, nervousness,
ataxia, nausea and vomiting, irritability, lethargy,
abdominal pain, pulse changes, constipation,
coordination problems

**Special Nursing Considerations
and Patient Education**
- Administer with food to decrease GI discomfort.
- Evaluate sleep patterns prior to therapy.
- Restrict amount of medication available because
  of possible dependence.
- Discontinue medication gradually.
- Provide safety measures (e.g., bedrails, handrails,
  call light).
- Monitor mental status.
- Inform patient that therapeutic effects may take 2
  nights.
- Provide alternate methods for sleep/relaxation:
  backrub, reading, exercises, relaxation breathing.
- Teach patient to
  - avoid alcohol and OTC medications.
  - report changes in sedation to physician.
  - avoid driving.

Trifluoperazine HCl

Brand Name
Stelazine

Actions
Antipsychotic, tranquilizer. Onset evident in 1–2 hours.

Uses
Schizophrenia

Contraindications
Meds Alcohol
Other Blood disorders, bone-marrow disorders, children under 16 unless hospitalized, hepatic impairment. *Use with caution:* Angina, epilepsy, glaucoma, parkinsonism, peptic ulcer, prostatic hypertrophy, respiratory disorder

Interactions
Amphetamines, antacids, anticonvulsants, antidepressants, antidiarrheals, antihistamine, atropine-like medications, CNS depressants, guanethidine, hypnotics, levodopa, MAO inhibitors, narcotics, phenytoin, quinidine, sedatives.

Dose
Adult PO: Initial dose: 1–5 mg bid; usual dose: 15–20 mg/day; *maximum* dose: 40 mg/day

370

Peds   PO: 6–12 yr (hospitalized): 1 mg qd–bid

Forms
Concentrate, Injection, tablets

Adverse Effects
Agitation, blurred vision, constipation, dizziness,
drowsiness, dry mouth, extrapyramidal symptoms,
hypotension, nasal congestion, tachycardia

**Special Nursing Considerations
and Patient Education**
- Protect medication from direct light.
- Dilute concentrate per manufacturer's instructions.
- Administer IM dose slowly into large muscle
  mass; keep patient in recumbent position for ½
  hour after administration.
- Monitor for fine vermicular tongue movements
  (may indicate early tardive dyskinesia).
- Offer hard candy (regular or sugar-free) to relieve
  dry mouth.
- When discontinued, decrease dosage gradually.
- Teach patient
  - that medication may cause photosensitivity and
    may discolor urine.
  - to be cautious when driving or involved in
    potentially hazardous tasks.
  - to use caution in hot weather and during
    strenuous exercise because of their impact on
    circulation.
  - to increase fluid and bulk intake.
  - to change position slowly.
  - to notify physician if any adverse effects occur.

Trihexyphenidyl HCl

Brand Name
Artane

Actions
Anticholinergic, antidyskinetic, muscle relaxant;
affects parasympathetic system. Onset evident in
1 hour.

Uses
Extrapyramidal disorders from CNS medications,
parkinsonism

Contraindications
Arteriosclerosis, children. *Use with caution:*
Glaucoma, myasthenia gravis, obstructive
disease of the GU or GI tract, prostatic
hypertrophy

Interactions
Alcohol, antacids, antidiarrheals, antihistamines,
antimuscarinics, barbiturates, CNS depressants,
haloperidol, MAO inhibitors, phenothiazines,
primidone, procainamide, quinidine, tricyclic
antidepressants

Dose
Adult   Individualized; initial dose: 1 mg/day;
increase to 6–10 mg/day in divided doses

372

Forms
Elixir, sustained-release capsules, tablets

Adverse Effects
Blurred vision, constipation, dizziness, drowsiness, dry mouth, insomnia, nausea, nervousness, urinary retention

Special Nursing Considerations and Patient Education
- Protect medication from direct light.
- Monitor vital signs until dosage is adjusted.
- Offer hard candy (regular or sugar-free) to relieve dry mouth.
- When discontinued, decrease dosage gradually.
- Be aware that
  - tolerance can develop.
- Teach patient to
  - not chew, crush, or break substained-release capsules.
  - take with meals to decrease gastric upset.
  - not take any nonprescription cough or hay fever preparations.
  - be cautious when driving or involved in potentially hazardous tasks.
  - use caution in hot weather and during strenuous exercise as medication may suppress perspiration.
  - increase fluid and bulk intake to decrease constipation.
  - notify physician for eye pain.

Trimethobenzamide HCl

Brand Name
Tigan

Actions
Antiemetic; inhibits medulla's chemoreceptor trigger zone. Onset evident in 20–40 minutes.

Uses
Nausea, vomiting

Contraindications
Meds Alcohol, CNS depressants
Other Benzocaine hypersensitivity, children (IM route), CNS depression, neonates and premature infants (suppositories). *Use with caution:* Allergies to antihistamines, dehydration, electrolyte imbalance, encephalitides, fever, gastroenteritis, Reye's syndrome

Interactions
Alkaloids derived from belladonna, barbiturates, phenothiazines, sedatives

Dose
Adult PO: 250 mg tid–qid
Peds Under 66 kg: (PO, rectal), 100 mg tid–qid
66–198 kg: (PO, rectal) 100–200 mg tid–qld

Forms
Capsules, injection, pediatric suppositories,
suppositories, tablets

Adverse Effects
Blurred vision, depression, diarrhea, disorientation, dizziness, drowsiness, dry mouth,
extrapyramidal symptoms, headache, hypotension, jaundice, muscle cramps

**Special Nursing Considerations
and Patient Education**
- Administer IM dose deep in upper, outer quadrant
  of gluteal muscle.
- Monitor blood pressure per physician's guidelines.
- Store suppositories in refrigerator.
- Be aware that
  - medication is administered to children only for
    prolonged vomiting with unknown etiology.
  - medication may mask toxic levels of other
    medications.
- Teach patient to
  - change position slowly to decrease
    hypotension.
  - be cautious when driving or involved in
    potentially hazardous tasks.
  - notify physician if rash, sore throat, or fever
    occur.

Vasopressin

Brand Name
Pitressin Tannate

Actions
Antidiuretic, posterior pituitary hormone, vasoconstrictor; aids in reabsorption of water in renal nephrons

Uses
Diabetes insipidus, gaseous distention

Contraindications
Angina, arteriosclerosis, chronic nephritis with nitrogen retention, ischemic heart disease, PVCs; IV route. *Use with caution:* Asthma, cardiac failure, children, migraine headache, vascular disease

Interactions
Acetaminophin, antidiabetic agents, diuretics, gangleonic blocking agents, heparin, lithium

Dose
Adult   Individualized; IM, SC 5–10 U 2–8x/day
Peds   Individualized

Forms
Injection

Adverse Effects
Circumoral pallor, dysrhythmias, hypersensitivity, MI, water intoxication

Special Nursing Considerations and Patient Education
* Before giving first dose, establish baseline data on patient's alertness, blood pressure, orientation, I&O, weight; recheck periodically throughout therapy.
* Monitor specific gravity and serum osmolality of patient's urine.
* Monitor lassess edema.
* Observe forsigns of water intoxication: behavior changes, disorientation, lethargy, neuromuscular excitability.
* Teach patient
  - to monitor urine specific gravity and serum osmolality at home per physician's guidelines.

Verapamil HCl

Brand Name
Calan, Isoptin

Actions
Antidysrhythmic, calcium antagonist; hinders calcium movement into select cardiovascular cells. Onset evident: IV 2–5 minutes; PO 30 minutes.

Uses
Paroxysmal supraventricular tachycardia, Prinzmetal's angina pectoris

Contraindications
Meds Beta-adrenergic blocking medications (given IV), calcium, disopyramide

Other Cardiogenic shock, 2nd or 3rd degree AV block, severe congestive heart failure, severe hypotension

Interactions
Antihypertensives, digitalis, highly protein-bound medications, quinidine

Dose
Adult IV bolus: initial dose, 5–10 mg; 10 mg 30 minutes later, PO 240–480 mg/day in divided doses

Peds   Under 1 yr: 0.1–0.2 mg/kg over 2 min;1–15
yr: 0.1–0.3 mg/kg over 2 min; repeat dose
after 30 min if necessary; *maximum* single
dose 10 mg

Forms
Solution (injection), tablets

Adverse Effects
Bradycardia, constipation, dizziness, edema,
headache, hypotension, nausea, tachycardia

Special Nursing Considerations
and Patient Education
- Monitor blood pressure before and after giving
  medication to evaluate patient's response.
- Monitor via a cardiac monitor during IV
  administration.
- Keep emergency equipment readily available.
- Monitor I&O,weight.
- Teach patient
  - to change position slowly to decrease
    hypotension.
  - to be cautious when driving or involved in
    potentially hazardous tasks.
  - take pulse prior to medication; notify physician if
    less than 50 bpm.

Warfarin Sodium

Brand Name
  Coumadin, Panwarfin

Actions
  Anticoagulant; hinders synthesis of prothrombin.
  Onset evident in 12 hours.

Uses
  Adjunct for coronary occlusion; atrial fibrillation
  with embolization, prophylactic use in pulmonary
  or venous thrombosis

Contraindications

Meds Alcohol, anesthetics

Other Blood dyscrasias, hemorrhagic tendency,
      hepatic or renal disease, malignant hyper-
      tension, peptic ulcer, polyarthritis, surgery,
      threatened abortion, ulcerative colitis,
      vitamin C deficiency. *Use with caution:*
      Allergies, anaphylactic disorders, diabetes,
      hepatic or renal insufficiency, infectious
      diseases, moderate to severe hypertension,
      polycythemia vera, vitamin K deficiency

Interactions
  Allopurinol, anabolic drugs, androgenic anabolic
  steroids, androgens, antacids, antibiotics, antidepressants, antihistamines, barbiturates, benzodi-

azepines, carbamazepine, chloral hydrate, chloramphenicol, chlorpromazine, cholestyramine, cortisone, coumarin, digitalis, disulfiram, d-thyroxine, estrogens, ethacrynic acid, glucagon, glutethimide, griseofulvin, haloperidol, hydroxyzine, indomethacin, insulin, isoniazid, mefenamic acid, mercaptopurine, methyldopa, methylphenidate, nalidixic acid, nortriptyline, oral contraceptives, oxyphenbutazone, para-aminosalicylic acid, phenylbutazone, phenylpropanolamine, phenyramidal, probenecid, propylthiouracil, quinidine, reserpine, salicylates, sulfinpyrazone, sulfonamides, sulfonylureas, thyroid preparations, tolbutamide NOTE: Oral anticoagulants have a greater potential for significant interactions than any other class of drugs.

Dose
Adult PO: initial dose, 40–60 mg, depending upon prothrombin times; *maintenance* dose: 2–10 mg/day depending upon prothrombin times

Forms
Injection, tablets

Adverse Effects
Abdominal cramps, anorexia, dermatitis, diarrhea, hemorrhage, nausea, urticaria, vomiting

**Special Nursing Considerations
and Patient Education**
- Protect medication from direct light.
- Administer medications exactly as ordered.
- Administer as a single daily dose unless ordered otherwise.
- Monitor prothrombin times.
- Do not change patient's diet because of possible impact on drug's effectiveness.
- When discontinued, decrease dosage gradually.
- Teach patient
  - that medication may discolor urine to orange.
  - to carry some type of Medic Alert card or bracelet.
  - to not take any other medications without notifying physician.
  - to notify physician of illness or any signs of hemorrhage.
  - to use soft toothbrush and electric razor to decrease possibility of hemorrhage.
  - if having dental work done, to inform dentist about this medication.

Part II

Appendices

Appendix A
Abbreviations

ACTH	Adrenocorticotropic hormone
ac	Before meals
AM	Morning
amps	Ampules
APTT	Activated partial thromboplastin time
ASAP	As soon as possible
AV	Atrioventricular
Avg.	Average
Bid	Twice a day
BUN	Blood urea nitrogen
CBC	Complete blood count
cc	Cubic centimeter
cm^2	Square centimeter
CNS	Central nervous system
CVA	Cerebral vascular accident
CVP	Central venous pressure
d	Day
D/C	Discontinue
DNA	Deoxyribonucleic acid
ECT	Electric convulsion therapy
EKG	Electrocardiogram
GI	Gastrointestinal
gm	Gram
gtt	Drops
GU	Genitourinary
h	Hour
hs	Hour of sleep

IM	Intramuscular
I&O	Intake and output
IV	Intravenous
KCl	Potassium chloride
kg	Kilogram
kg/min	Kilogram per minute
m^2	Square meter
MAO	Monoamine oxidase (MAO inhibitor)
mEq	Milliequivalent; one-thousandth of an equivalent or specific weighted measurement
Mg	Magnesium
μg	Microgram
mg	Milligram
MI	Myocardial infarction
min	Minute
ml	Milliliter
mm^3	Cubic millimeter
OTC	Over the counter
PO	By mouth
PC	After meals
PM	Afternoon
prn	As needed
PTT	Partial thromboplastin time
PVC	Premature ventricular contraction
q	Every
qd	Every day
qid	Four times a day
qod	Every other day
RNA	Ribonucleic acid
SC	Subcutaneous
tid	Three times a day
U	Units
WBC	White blood cells

Appendix B
Side Effect Groupings

Allergic reactions
- Delayed: angioedema, arthralgia, fever, lymph-adenopathy, splenomegaly
- Mild: angioedema, asthma, cramping (abdominal), diarrhea, dizziness, drowsiness, dyspepsia, fever, headache, hives, nausea, pruritis, rash, rhinitis, tinnitus, vomiting
- Severe: bone-marrow depression, confusion, extrapyramidal symptoms, fatigue, high fever, hallucinations, hemorrhage, hepatitis, jaundice, joint pains, palpitations, sore throat, weakness

Androgenic effects: breast-size reduction, hirsutism, voice deepening

Drug fever: ataxia, blurred vision, dizziness, irritability, numbness and tingling (circumoral/peripheral), weakness

Ergotism: confusion, diarrhea, dizziness, headache, nausea, vomiting

Extrapyramidal symptoms: akathisia, dystonia, parkinsonism, tardive dyskinesia

Hyperglycemia: excessive hunger and thirst, excessive urination, headache, nausea, positive urinary glucose and ketones, pulse increase, sweet-smelling breath, weight loss

Hyperkalemia: areflexia, breathing difficulty, confusion, parethesias, weakness

386

Hypoglycemia: anxiety, diaphoresis, drowsiness, fatigue, headache, lassitude, nausea, tremulousness

Hypokalemia: anorexia, confusion, hypotension, lethargy, muscle weakness, nausea

Hyponatremia: abdominal cramps, drowsiness, dry mouth, lethargy, thirst

Hypertensive crisis: increasing confusion, rapid increase in blood pressure, vision changes

Lupus erythematosus syndrome: arthritis, fever, myalgia, pleuritic pain, polyarthralgia, skin lesions

Nephrotoxicity: albuminuria, hematuria, retention of nitrogen, urinary casts

Ototoxicity: deafness, dizziness, sense of fullness in the ears, tinnitus, vertigo

Renal failure: albuminuria, azotemia, cylinduria

Thrombosis: chest/leg pain, respiratory distress

Uremia: drowsiness, foul breath, headache, lethargy restlessness, vomiting

Appendix C
Nursing Interventions for
Common Side Effects

Bone-marrow suppression
- Observe for signs and symptoms of infection, i.e., slow healing wound with inflammation, swelling and/or discharge or a cold that does not get better.
- Observe any abnormal bleeding tendencies: i.e., increased bruising, petechiae, frequent nosebleeds, bleeding from gums.
- Brush teeth with toothettes or clean with gauze; avoid hard toothbrushes.
- Apply pressure for several minutes over injection sites.
- Observe changes in activity level and physical appearance for anemia, i.e., lethargy, fatigability, pallor of the skin and mucous membranes, dyspnea, heart palpitations.

Constipation
- Increase intake of foods high in fiber.
- Increase intake of water and other fluids.
- Include more fresh vegetables and fruits in the diet.

388

- Do not utilize laxatives unless directed to do so by the physician.

Nausea
- Keep dry carbohydrate foods at the bedside (dry crackers or toast). Eat a small amount before getting out of bed.
- Eat small frequent meals rather than three large meals.
- Monitor diet and eliminate those foods that aggravate the nausea.
- Do not utilize medications unless directed to do so by the physician.

Orthostatic hypotension
- When the patient is getting out of bed:
  - Have a chair or other support near the bedside.
  - Sit up slowly.
  - Dangle legs and feet over the side of the bed for several minutes.
  - Slowly stand up, sitting down if any dizziness occurs.
- When the patient is standing up from a chair:
  - Move to the edge of the chair slowly.
  - Sit there for a few minutes.
  - Slowly stand up, sitting down if any dizziness occurs.
  - Utilize a side chair or other support to stand up.

Appendix D
Conversion Information

APOTHECARY SYSTEM TO METRIC SYSTEM
(WEIGHT)

gr xv	= 1.0	gm =	1000	mg
gr x	= 0.6	gm =	600	mg
gr viiss (ss=$1/2$)	= 0.5	gm =	500	mg
gr v	= 0.3	gm =	300	mg
gr iii	= 0.2	gm =	200	mg
gr 1-$1/2$	= 0.1	gm =	100	mg
gr 1	= 0.06	gm =	60	mg
gr $3/4$	= 0.05	gm =	50	mg
gr $1/2$	= 0.03	gm =	30	mg
gr $1/4$	= 0.015	gm =	15	mg
gr $1/6$	= 0.010	gm =	10	mg
gr $1/8$	= 0.008	gm =	8	mg
gr $1/12$	= 0.005	gm =	5	mg
gr $1/15$	= 0.004	gm =	4	mg
gr $1/20$	= 0.0032	gm =	3	mg
gr $1/30$	= 0.0022	gm =	2	mg
gr $1/40$	= 0.0015	gm =	1.5	mg
gr $1/50$	= 0.0012	gm =	1.2	mg
gr $1/60$	= 0.001	gm =	1	mg
gr $1/100$	= 0.0006	gm =	0.6	mg
gr $1/120$	= 0.0005	gm =	0.5	mg
gr $1/150$	= 0.0004	gm =	0.4	mg
gr $1/200$	= 0.0003	gm =	0.3	mg
gr $1/300$	= 0.0002	gm =	0.2	mg
gr $1/600$	= 0.0001	gm =	0.1	mg

METRIC SYSTEM TO APOTHECARY SYSTEM

Weight

0.06	gm =	1	grain
1	gm =	15	grains
4	gm =	1	dram
30	gr =	1	ounce
1	kg =	2.2	pounds

Volume

0.06	ml =	1	minim
1	ml =	15	minims
4	ml =	1	fluidram
30	ml =	1	fluidounce
500	ml =	1	pint
1000	ml =	1	quart

Appendix E
General Guidelines for the
Administration of Medications

Exercise caution when administering any medication to:

- Children
- Debilitated individuals
- Drug dependent individuals
- Elderly individuals
- Lactating females
- Pregnant females
- Individuals anticipating immediate surgery

Exercise caution when administering any medication to an individual for the first time.

Administration of any medication to an individual who previously experienced an allergic or hypersensitive reaction is contraindicated.

Remind patients to

- Take medications exactly as directed.
- Check dates on all medications prior to taking.
- Not discontinue a medication without conferring with the physician.

Available information on a medication is not indicative of the level of safety for that medication.

Excretion of medication occurs through the intestines, kidneys, liver, lungs or skin, and impairment of these organs indicates the need for caution when administering medications.

Advise patients to complete the regimen of medications that has been ordered even if they no longer feel ill.

Crushing an enteric coated or sustained-release capsule/tablet is contraindicated. Mixing the contents of sustained-release capsules for administration is contraindicated.

Include discharge teaching for any medications which the patient will be taking at home.

Review the patient's current medications when administering a new medication to avoid any problematic interactions.

Advising patients to be "cautious" indicates that they will experience some impairment in their normal levels of functioning.

Appendix F
Food Groups

- *Potassium-rich:* Almonds, apricots, bananas, beans (lima, navy), beef, chicken, citrus fruits, coconut, dates, dried figs, fish, lentils, melons, milk, orange juice, peaches, peanut butter, raw carrots, rye crackers
- *Tyramine-rich:* Avocados, bananas, beverages (from meat/yeast extracts), broad beans, caffeine, cheese, chicken, chocolate, figs, licorice, liver, meat tenderizer, pickled herring, raisins, sour cream, soy sauce, unpasteurized beer, vermouth, wine (chianti), yeast extracts, yogurt
- *High Fat:* Bacon, bologna, butter, butter rolls, butter crackers, cheese, 4% fat cottage chese, corn chips, cream, croissants, doughnuts, frankfurters, gravy with meat drippings, heavily marbled meats, ice cream, lard, milk (whole or 2%), oil-packed tuna, pastrami, potato chips, salad dressings, salami, sausage, sour cream, whole eggs, whole milk cheeses
- *Cholesterol High: Beef, butter, caviar, cheese (cream, 25–30%, cheddar), crab meat, egg yolk, heart, kidney, lard, lobster, milk (whole), oysters, shrimp, sweetbreads, veal*
- *Cholesterol Low:* Breads, buttermilk, cereals, cottage cheese, fruits, lean meat and fish, skim or non-fat milk, vegetables (without butter, cream, lard), vegetable oil and vegetable oil margarine
- *Gluten-free:* Corn flour, cornmeal, cornstarch, gluten-free wheat starch, gluten-free bread mix, lima bean flour, potato flour, rice flour, soy flour

References

Adrenergics (sympathomimetics). (1983). *Nursing 83, 13*(1), 64a–64b.

Albanese, J. (1979). Nurses' *Drug Reference*. New York: McGraw-Hill.

Aminoglycosides. (1983). *Nursing 83, 13* (2), 64a–64b.

Antianxiety agents. (1983). *Nursing 83, 13* (4), 64a–64b.

Antihypertensives. (1983). *Nursing 83, 13* (3), 64a–64b.

Armstrong, M., Dickason, E., Howe, J., Jones, D. & Snider, M. (Eds.).
(1979). *McGraw-Hill Handbook of Clinical Nursing.* New York: McGraw-Hill.

Bergersen, B. & Goth, A. (1977). *Pharmacology in Nursing,* (14th Ed.) St. Louis: Mosby.

Brooks, S. (Ed.). (1978). *Nurses, Drug Reference.* Boston: Little, Brown.

Deglin, J., and Vallerand, A. (1988). *Davis's Drug Guide for Nurses.* Philadelphia: F.A. Davis.

Govoni, L. & Hayes, J. (1982). *Drugs and Nursing Implications.* New York: Appleton-Century-Crofts.

Hussar, D.,PhD. (1982). New Drugs. *Nursing 82, 12* (5),34.

Karch, A. & Boyd, E. (1989). *Handbook of Drugs and the Nursing Process.* Philadelphia: J.B. Lippincott.

Kirilloff, L. & Libbals, S. (1983). Drugs for asthma: a complete guide. *American Journal of Nursing. 83,* 55–61.

395

Loebl, S., Spratto, G. & Heckheimer, E. (1980). *The Nurse's Drug Handbook,* (2nd ed.). New York: Wiley.

Long, J. (1977). *The Essential Guide to Prescription Drugs: What You Need to Know for Safe Drug Use.* New York: Harper & Row.

Nurses' drug alert. (1982). *American Journal of Nursing, 82* (7), 1121–1128.

Nurses' drug alert. (1982). *American Journal of Nursing, 82* (9), 1425–1432.

Nurses' drug alert. (1982). *American Journal of Nursing, 82* (11),1749–1756.

Nursing 81 Drug Handbook. (1981). Horsham, PA: Intermed Communications.

Penicillins. (1983). *Nursing 83, 13* (6), 64a–64b.

Physicians' Desk Reference. (1989). (43rd ed.). Oradell,N.J.: Medical Economics Co.

Skidmor-Roth, L. (1990). *Mosby's Nursing Drug Reference.* St. Louis: C.V. Mosby.

Thrombolytic enzymes. (1983). *Nursing 83,* 13 (5), 64a–64b.

US Pharmacopial Convention. (1980). *United States Dispensing Information 1980.* Easton, PA: Mack Printing Company.

Wiener, M., Pepper, A., Kuhn-Weisman, G. & Romano, J. (1979). *Clinical Pharmacology and Therapeutics in Nursing.* New York: McGraw-Hill.

Wordell, D. (1982). Should you crush that tablet? *Nursing 82, 12* (9),78.

Generic Index

397

398

Brand Name

A-poxide, 68
AK-Mycin, 146
ASA, 36
Achromycin, 348
Actifed, 322
Adapin, 140
Advil, 192
Aerobid, 156
Aldactone, 336
Aldoclor, 70
Aldomet, 238
Alupent, 234
Amen, 228
Amicar, 16
Amoxil, 28
Amytal, 26
Anaprox, 256
Anaprox, 258
Ansaid, 162
Armour Thyroid, 356
Artane, 372
Atarax, 190
Ativan, 222
Atrovent, 204
Augmentin, 30
Aventyl, 270
Bactrim, 100
Benadryl, 134
Benylin, 10
Benylin, 134
Bethaprim, 100
Betoptic, 48
Biocadrea, 358
Brevital, 236

Bumex, 50
Buspar, 52
Butisol, 54
Calan, 378
Capoten, 56
Cardizem, 130
Catapres, 92
Ceclor, 60
Ceftin, 62
Cerebid, 280
Cerespan, 280
Chlorazine, 314
Cin-Quin, 324
Cipro, 84
Cleocin, 88
Clinoril, 338
Clonopin, 90
Cogentin, 46
Combipres, 92
Comoxol, 100
Compazine, 314
Corafate, 334
Corganol, 252
Corgard, 252
Cotrim, 100
Coumadin, 380
Crystodigin, 126
Curretab, 228
Dalmane, 160
Darvon, 318
Datril, 2
Decadron, 114
Declomycin, 106
Deltasone, 310

Systems Index

407

408

410

Made in the USA
Middletown, DE
31 May 2023

31790462R00236